SIRTFOOD DIET
cookbook

Easy, delicious, and healthy recipes
to activate your skinny gene.

With a 7-day meal plan
to start losing weight right now!

Kate Adkins

Table of Contents

Chapter 6. Breakfast Recipes 49

Chapter 7. Juice Recipes 62

Chapter 8. Smoothie Recipes 71

Introduction

Being healthy and losing weight is an everyday choice. You have to take those first baby steps and see how it can change you and your life.

If you want to reap the amazing results of Sirtfoods, here is some suggested ways to jumpstart your diet:

- **Safety first** - Before starting any particular diet or regimen, consult your healthcare provider especially if you have an existing illnesses. This will ensure that the diet will not sabotage any medications that you might be taking or have an adverse effect to your health. Do not worry, the Sirtfood diet is fairly safe.

- **Knowledge is power** - This diet is still bran new, but there is still a good amount of information available and more upcoming since this diet is fast gaining popularity. In addition, you can also search the internet for recipes, food alternatives, nutrient content and more.

- **Follow the guidelines** - Sirtfood is guaranteed to bring results, if and only if you carefully follow the diet guide and suggested food.

- **Help yourself** - Aside from following what is allowed in the food program, you can start by eliminating processed and starchy food from your normal diet. Stop eating junk! This will fast track the result of Sirtfood Diet.

- **Start a physical activity** - Sirtfood diet can indeed burn those fats and build muscle, but I recommend that you start adding physical activities to your daily routine. A 30-minute walk a day would do wonders to your body and will also fast track the results. In addition, there are many wonderful effects when exercising like: preventing and combating health conditions, helping improve your mood, promoting better sleep, burning calories, giving you an energy boost and more.

- **Hit the supermarket** - The Sirtfood diet depends on certain foods. These foods were chosen because of their sirtuin-triggering ability. So if you do not follow the list, well, you won't see results. Do not worry, because I will be providing list of suggested foods; Plus there are no overly expensive type of foods and you can find it readily available almost anywhere.

- **Be ready with the initial "restrictions"** - Of course, if you want to see different results, you have to "sacrifice" a little in order to achieve the full benefits of the Sirtfood diet. But don't worry, the first three days are only the hardest ones for this diet since there will be calorie restrictions involved, but rest assured that it will become easier each day. Although for others who tried the diet, the restrictions set was not that hard for them, the reason is careful planning of meals. Plan your meals ahead - Whatever diet you may be on, planning your meals is a big help. Not only will it reduce the stress from dieting, you can also have the chance to weigh your choices and fill in your cupboard. For the first phase of this diet, you have to follow a calorie count. You will be surprised that there are many filling dishes allowed with less calories and packed with sirtuins.

- **Involve a diet partner** - This diet could also greatly benefit your family, partner or friends, plus it is easier when you have an accountability partner to remind you, share recipes with or even cook dishes with.

- **Document your progress** - You can start by taking "before" pictures and take necessary body measurements. You could also keep a food diary so that you can watch your food intake. Observe the changes in your body with each week or phase. You can also have a set of goals to further push you to continue with the diet.

- **Be kind to yourself** - Do not set too high expectations. Yes, some can easily lose 7 pounds in a week, but remember that our bodies are not all the same; and of course your level of commitment will also count. Other variables could be adding of an exercise regimen in the diet plan, which could make the losing weight process faster.

Chapter 1
The Real Health Sirtfoods

The Health Benefits

There is proof that sirtuin activators may provide a wide variety of health benefits as well as muscle strengthening and appetite suppression. That involves having better memory, better control of blood sugar levels in the body, and the clearance of damage caused by free radical molecules that build up in cells and result in cancer and other diseases.

"The positive effects of the intake of food and beverages rich in sirtuin activators in decreasing chronic disease risk are important observational evidence," said Professor Frank Hu, an authority on diet and epidemiology at Harvard University in a recent paper in Advances In Nutrition. An anti-ageing diet is particularly suited to a Sirt food diet.

While the entire plant realm is home to sirtuin activators, only some fruits and vegetables have enough to report as Sirtfood. Examples include green tea, cacao powder, Indian spice pea, spinach, onion and parsley.

In many stores, fruit and vegetables such as strawberries, avocados, bananas, spinach, kiwis, broccoli, and pep are actually quite low activators for sirtuins. This does not mean, however, that they are not worth eating because they have many other advantages.

The advantage of a Sirtfood-packed diet is that it's much more versatile than other diets. You could just consume a few Sirt foods healthily. Or you could concentrate on them. The 5:2 diet could require more calories on low-calorie days by incorporating Sirt foods.

One notable observation of a Sirtfood diet trial is that participants lose excessive weight without weakening their muscles. It was also normal for participants to build weight, contributing to a more formed and toned body. It is the beauty of Sirtfoods: fat burning is activated, but muscle growth, maintenance and repair are promoted as well. In comparison to other foods, weight reduction typically occurs from fat and muscle, which slows down the digestion of the body and allows weight to rebound more easily.

Are there any other benefits of Sirtfoods?

Sirtuins have a hand in several other safe advantages as well. Including:

Sleep

Activating sirtuins adds to improving of the circadian cycle such that you generate hormones while you improve your sleep cycle.

Diabetes

Sirtuins allow cells to be more responsive to insulin so that they can lose more blood glucose. As the key to both diabetes and weight gain is insulin resistance, there can be positive news for the waistline.

Memory

Turmeric boosts short-term performance and defends against cognitive disorders. Pack your morning juice to begin the day more brainy.

Lean Gene

Genetics is a long-standing beat-up cause. This is why people are lazy, weak, and behave as though they do not realize what's going on in their lives. Yeah, certain mutations may render you predisposed to a disease, but that does not indicate that must have it as you get older. You can also ensure that you grow good genes in life by not building poor habits. It means that you can build as strong an atmosphere as you can to prevent inherited vulnerabilities.

It appears like biology is the direction in which our scientific world shifts. This is terrifying. Essentially, our chromosomes are what creates us. If we fix the right genetic code somewhere, we could all be the same. There has been a lot of talk about tests in mice and the consequences of "obesity mutation." They want to see why people are fat.

The obesity gene was long known, but just recently, how this gene functions was revealed. We named the FTO mutation, and mice who had not pigged the mutation were slouched all day long and miraculously appeared more healthy. It seems like the right cure for individuals to do or feed properly. Any other study has shown that individuals with this amazing FTO gene have an excess of 7 pounds heavier and 70% more likely to be obese. 70% is a big amount. Either we have individuals who will not want to remain alive, or this gene is just an end to all genes. My guess is that people don't want to remain safe.

Mice are really similar to us when it comes to our genes and DNA, and the experiments performed on this mouse will demonstrate how we accumulate any extra weight from this FTO mutation. To pharmaceutical firms, this is a fairly major move. Their number has projected about 400 million obese people in the world and its rising. Here in states, for every three men, 2 of them are overweight. These figures are bad, but they get worse. This indicates that something about the program is incorrect. All this needs to be changed.

Being obese raises any risk factor that you could think about. If you have to bear this additional weight, your body faces a lot more pain than normal. Imagine wearing a dumbbell weighing around 50 pounds anywhere you go.

Such studies will ultimately contribute to obesity care. They view obesity as a disorder and not as a preference for lifestyle. People may lose weight; the FTO gene may or may not be lost. Some will consider it difficult, but it is always feasible. I can see the future. I will see the future. When the first advert on television speaks about the consequences of the FTO mutation, they inquire if you are fat with certain alarming figures, then comes the main selling advertisement on whatever the medication is.

This is my pet peeve. Why do we investigate this? Yeah, for the sake of information, it is necessary and can be achieved, but why not look to the past where the citizens were not fat? See how slim they were, what they were drinking and how they were sleeping. We will avoid researching illness here in pursuit of wellness—health research to determine fitness. Look at mature cultures that were generally healthy. Look at how strong and slim they were.

So, my aim is to avoid researching illness in order to pursue wellness. Do not allow your chromosomes to dictate who you are and how you are. Your climate and biology play an important role, and I think it plays a more important role than we think. You have the opportunity to improve yourself, whether it be autism, a professional athlete, succeeding in school or some other reason. You should do it, whether it's healthy genes or not.

Do You Have Lean Genes?

What is your genetic weight? Just 5% of all weight disorders compensate for obesity genes. About 95% of the weight issues are due to chromosomes. This fact has not affected our culture's high incidence of obesity. Nor should we blame the issue of obesity on high-fat diets. Because fat contains nine calories per gram, unlike the carbs or protein that only contain four calories per gram, our crisis still cannot be nailed to fat consumption. Evidence has demonstrated, in addition, that low-fat diets do not work well and do more damage than good. And to add to that –avoiding fat in your diet is not a major determinant of body fat. The Women's Wellness Project, the first diet and body weight research study, showed that 50,000 people have no substantial loss of weight in low-fat diets.

But without the specific check – the main way to avoid slipping into the 'skinny-fat' group is a full and healthy diet. Here's a trick - because you have a higher rating, you will consume better. Meaning, if you have more lean muscle mass than fat to sustain your weight, you will potentially consume more. Your body is a robotic oven that can break down everything you consume quickly – and comfortably. Not that it all burns down quickly. If you consume unhealthy foods into your body, your muscle mass reduces, and the capacity to lose calories is therefore reduced. There are two main things that improve lean muscle mass - exercise resistance and protein. Both inappropriate proportions for your body type and your workout intensity should give you the perfect fat - lean muscle ratio.

Turning to the topic of obesity and weight care, the main aspect is to personalize the strategy. We learn more and more about something named Nutri-genomics in my area of agriculture. It is the awareness of how we can affect our genes through food. Yeah, this has been learned - our diet will affect and probably alter the expression of our genome. If you like, let's name it Genetic Eating. When we supply the body with building blocks and good nutrients, the genes "turn on" as it were. Put simply - you come into this world with some genetic make-up, and if you do not properly "feed" your genes-the healthy expression of those genes are stopped. For example, let us refer to it as the "good weight gene" without the proper nutrients, this gene shuts down. To switch the genetic light on, we will need to send our body the correct current (a little wordplay) – for it to work. This is, in reality, a very basic description for a very complicated operation. The most important aspect you can realize is that you should adjust your DNA to blend in with your clothes, so YOUR Food is one of the most important functions.

7-Day Meal Plan

The truth behind the seven-day eating plan that claims to strip away weight. The diet promises to torch fat within a week, while leaving intact muscle. But there's more to Sirtfoods than miraculous promises–if the evidence behind it is working out, it might show that we've been talking about eating healthy the wrong way for decades.

One way or another, you've heard of the Sirt Diet, even if you don't recognize the name. It is described as the kilo-shredding program in news reports that encourages you to eat chocolate and drink red wine, pledging to look like a supermodel and behave like a superhero.

But the fact is, behind Sirt there is much more analytical clout than the usual drop-fat-fast scheme. It is based on a family of compounds which have only been found in the past decade, and experimental evidence shows that they are much more significant than formerly thought. And if the people behind it are right, then when we're talking about what to eat we need to change our attention.

Days	Breakfast	Lunch	Dinner	Snack
Day 1	Hot Caramel Apple Juice	Delicious Green Juice	Shrimp and Endives	Fresh, Homemade Apple Juice
Day 2	Heavenly Honeydew Juice	Minty Tomatoes and Corn	Ginger-beet Juice	V-great Juice
Day 3	Delicious Green Juice	Fresh, Homemade Apple Juice	Tuna and Tomatoes	Heavenly Honeydew Juice
Day 4	Sirtfood Baked Breakfast Potatoes	Smothered Swai	V-great Juice	Delicious Green Juice
Day 5	Heavenly Honeydew Juice	Ginger Asian Slaw	Hot Caramel Apple Juice	Plum & Pistachio Snack
Day 6	Artichoke Eggs	V-great Juice	Fresh, Homemade Apple Juice	Kale Sauté
Day 7	Ginger-beet Juice	Delicious Green Juice	Cherry Chicken Lettuce Wraps	Mini Bagel Pizzas

Chapter 2
Health and Weight loss Benefits of Sirtfoods

Obesity

We all know that caloric restriction is one of the classic methods to induce weight loss. Countless studies have proven its effects. Yet, it is also well-known that for some people reducing calorie intake alone is not enough. Thankfully, when calorie reduction is paired with increased polyphenol intake, you can increase weight loss and combat obesity.

There are many stories of people losing a lot of weight on the Sirt diet, but Adele's stunning fifty-pound loss is the most well-known success story.

Obesity is currently known as a significant threat to the Western world, as it promotes disease, and it can be challenging to combat. Many people try all their lives to reach a healthy weight level but continue to struggle. This is mostly why over thirty percent of the United States population is clinically obese, with the condition affecting women to a more significant degree. But, if you, like Adele, can shed the pounds with the Sirt diet, not only will it be easier to shop for clothes and experience higher energy levels, you will also be able to reduce your risk of several weight-related chronic diseases.

Immune Health

We all know that the immune system is essential; you learn about it early on in school. However, most of us never consider our immune health until we get sick, and by then, it is already partly too late. Unless we come down with a cold, the flu, or worse, a disease of some sort, we give little thought to this vital part of the body. But, at this point, all our immune system can do is damage control, trying to fight off the infection so that it doesn't kill us instead. We would be much better off if we instead focused on immune health all of the time so that we can prevent these infections from occurring in the first place. Think about it, would you rather have to try to fight off the flu once you already have it, or avoid ever getting it in the first place? Of course, polyphenols can't take the place of vaccines, antibiotics, and other medicine. Still, they can significantly help you and strengthen both your immune system's ability to prevent infections and fight off ones you might come down with.

Heart Health

Oxidative stress, a leading cause for cellular aging, is a factor in both high blood pressure and heart diseases. Therefore, scientists in a 2004 study sought to learn if the polyphenols found in tea could help treat overall heart health by repairing and reducing oxidative stress. The results were encouraging, showing that when stroke-prone mice with high blood pressure consume either green or black tea, they can significantly lower both systolic and diastolic blood pressure. By the end of the study, the researchers concluded that the regular consumption of tea could protect against high blood pressure in humans.

Olives and extra virgin olive oil have long been known to have several positive health benefits, but this has mostly been attributed to the monounsaturated fats found within olives. A study published in 2006 sought to learn if all of the health claims were genuinely associated with the monounsaturated fat, or if the polyphenols found within extra virgin olive oil were contributing to the positive effects, as well. To test this, researchers administered three different types of olive oil to participants with varying levels of polyphenols within the oil. Suffice to say, extra virgin olive oil is the richest in polyphenols, and the more processed and refined a brand of olive oil is, the fewer polyphenols it will contain.

Stroke

Sometimes referred to as a brain attack, strokes are extremely dangerous. While it deals with blood and many of the same risk factors of heart disease can cause it, it is a separate category than cardiovascular health as it centers in the brain. What happens when a person has a stroke? A tear in a person's blood vessels or a blood clot results in the supply of blood to the brain is blocked off. There are two types of stroke. These are hemorrhagic and ischemic.

Thyroid Health

While we all frequently hear about the importance of heart, lung, stomach, and other organ health, the thyroid is commonly underappreciated by all but those who have a thyroid disorder. While it may not be a major organ, it is located at the base of the neck that manages the functioning of many of our organs. Your liver, kidneys, heart, brain, and even skin would be unable to function without it properly!

The thyroid is a gland and part of the endocrine system, which produces, stores, and releases hormones for the use of our cells. If it either under provides or overproduces these hormones, it results in several severe symptoms that worsen as they continue to get further away from homeostasis. Thyroid hormones manage systems such as:

- Heart Rate
- Breathing
- Body Weight
- Metabolism
- Cholesterol
- Body Temperature
- Muscle Strength
- Menstrual Cycle
- Central Nervous System
- Peripheral Nervous System

The good news is that a 2011 study found that polyphenols can improve thyroid function. It can do this in a few ways. This study focused on the effect of polyphenols that allow the thyroid to absorb more of the iodide it requires to produce hormones. However, this does not mean that if your thyroid already overproduces these hormones that it will worsen the problem, as the thyroid does not release all of the hormones it produces. Instead, it waits for the brain to signal it to release the formerly built and stored hormones before releasing them into the bloodstream. Simply put, it allows the thyroid to regain homeostasis.

Type II Diabetes

While polyphenols have long been underestimated, a study published as early as 2002 did analyze the effects of polyphenols from green tea on individuals with type II diabetes. This is excellent news, especially since type II diabetes is the most prevalent, and the number of people diagnosed only continues to rise. The results were incredibly successful, finding that these polyphenols can increase glucose tolerance and reduce serum glucose levels. Both of these effects were great, but they only improved and expanded over time as the rats consumed tea-based polyphenols on a more regular basis.

Another appraisal, this one published in 2015, has noted how several studies have shown that a diet rich in polyphenols has time and again proven to be a successful means to combat type II diabetes. This appraisal found that not only can polyphenols prevent this type of diabetes, it can also actively manage and treat the condition in many individuals. Some of the other benefits of polyphenols that help with diabetes include antioxidant and anti-inflammatory effects, protection of the pancreatic cells from glucose toxicity, decreased starch digestion, and more.

Kidney Health

Many people develop kidney (renal) disorders as they age, which is only worsened due to poor dietary habits, excessive alcohol, and other lifestyle factors. Thankfully, a 2007 scientific appraisal found that polyphenols can affect the kidneys from injury, increase antioxidant defenses, and keep the renal cells functioning in a desired state of homeostasis. This was especially helpful in diabetic patients who frequently develop diabetic nephropathy of the kidneys, which was lessened due to the polyphenols. Lastly, the study found that when participants drank red wine, the undesired effects that alcohol frequently has on blood pressure were counterbalanced in thanks to the protective elements of the polyphenols.

Autoimmune Disorders

There is a wide range of autoimmune disorders, over a hundred in total, which can all affect the body differently! This naturally means that the way polyphenols help each disease will vary. However, the good news is that polyphenols, in theory, should be able to help every type of autoimmune disorder.

The one aspect that all autoimmune disorders share is that they are affected by the immune system, hence the word "autoimmune." While the purpose of the immune system is to protect the body from infection and illness actively, this is disrupted when a person has an autoimmune disorder. When this happens, the immune system begins to attack a person's own body instead of invading bacteria or disease. By striking a person's healthy cells, the immune system damages these cells and causes a wide array of symptoms. But, by optimizing the immune system to attain a state of homeostasis, you can reduce the number of attacks caused by the disorder. Earlier, we explained how polyphenols help the immune system to maintain a state of homeostasis. Thus, polyphenols can also help to treat autoimmune diseases.

Several studies have successfully found polyphenols to treat both autoimmune disorders in general and specific autoimmune diseases. Some of these studies have tested type I diabetes, Sjogren's syndrome, myocarditis, thyroiditis, rheumatoid arthritis, and more!

Bone Health

It is incredibly important to protect your bone health, especially as you age. People frequently develop osteoporosis at an older age, which results in bone deterioration and bone mass loss. Both of these result in an increased risk of fractures and breaks, which is why many people begin to break more bones when they fall as they age. Not only should the elderly be concerned about this, as some people develop bone disorders at a younger age. People who have taken or have to take prescribed steroids regularly should be especially aware of the risks, as one of the most common adverse effects of steroids is bone deterioration.

Many people think that by drinking more milk, they can increase their bone health, but the truth is that studies have found dairy to be much less effective than other methods in raising bone density. For instance, multiple studies have found polyphenols to be especially helpful in increasing bone health overall and both preventing and treating osteoporosis.

Neurodegenerative Disorders

Many types of neurodegenerative disorders can affect people of all ages. However, the most common and worrying for most people is Alzheimer's disease, as we never know if it is a condition our loved ones or we will develop as we age. It is especially concerning, as Alzheimer's disease is only growing in prevalence each year, with forty-four million people worldwide living with the disease. Thankfully, we don't have to accept that Alzheimer's may simply be inevitable. While we might be unable to prevent it in all cases, studies have shown that by eating a diet rich in polyphenols, we can protect our brain health and significantly reduce our risk of developing this devastating condition.

If you hope to protect yourself from Alzheimer's disease, Parkinson's disease, or several other neurodegenerative disorders, there is study after study proving the positive effect polyphenols have in preventing and managing these conditions.

As you can see, there are a significant number of conditions that polyphenols can both help treat and prevent, by merely increasing your consumption of them. When you combine dietary increase of polyphenols with calorie restriction and healthy weight, you only improve your health further while decreasing your risk of injury and disease.

Chapter 3
Keto Diet and Sirtfood Diet

Let's get real. How can the human body have so many different ways of slimming it down?

There seems to be another new diet every year, which comes in the hot press with the approval of some great celebrities. It makes its big debut and thanks to every popular magazine on the check-out line in the food store. Another health expert who is part of a popular lecture show explains the science behind this new diet as if it were an entire discovery.

Nevertheless, you cannot help but wonder if this may be the trick to help you get back into your favorite jeans long before the children are born. Or at least before adulthood, sorry sweetheart said your days are over to eat whatever you want without getting a single pound.

There have been two diet plans over the last few years that have brought it to the fore. The low-carbon, fatty Keto diet and the "skinny gene" boost Sirtfood diet are available.

Hold up

What's the distinction between the two? What's best for your plans for health and weight loss? What is a "skinny gene" in the world?!

However, let us explore everything there is to know about each diet to answer your questions. This is your ultimate guide to everything behind them, the Sirt and the science.

What's the Keto Diet?

Let's continue with the diet keto, or ketogenic. In brief, a keto diet consists of a small consumption of starch, milk protein, and high-fat products. Real Keto peeps try to drink 20g or less of carbohydrates daily, most of which are consumed from healthy fat sources. Invented by Peter Huttenlocher back in the 1970s, the notion behind this is that our body is in a state of ketosis. What now? What now? This is another excellent way to say that your metabolism does not rely on glycogen and begins to relish fat for energy.

Your body (especially your liver) releases small molecules called ketones that act to offer your body energy. At the same time, our sugar levels are somewhat low if you reduce your carb and calorie intake.

Ketones are made from fat, so your body is reprogrammed to fat in contrast to glucose on this diet. By limiting your calorie consumption and, in some ways, exerting your body to relish fat for fuel, fat stores are accessible throughout your body when you need energy.

Looks reasonable, okay? Now, we're going to switch gears and talk SIRT!

What's Sirtfood Diet?

Before we know about the SIRT diet program, let us be mindful of the fact that this diet allows you to consume (in moderation) red wine and chocolate. How can that be?

This latest diet plan, established by nutritionists, means that many Sirt products are eaten. This means foods that produce a protein called Sirtuin in our body.

These particular small proteins help reduce inflammation and defend our cells against stress damage. Ah, so sirtuins are for cells as we have red wine. Everything's making sense!

Seriously, a Sirtfood diet will boost your metabolism and burn fat quickly. Men and women reported falling up to seven pounds a week after this diet plan had begun.

In contrast to the ketogenic diet, the diet is divided into two phases. You need to minimize your daily consumption to 1000-calories during the first three days while you have three green shirts- food juices plus one sirt-food meal daily.

Four to seven days, you can maximize your consumption to 1,500-calories while you enjoy 2-3 green juices and a Sirt meal a day. Then the next two weeks will be called the maintenance period, and your body will appear to be continuously losing weight.

This cycle is known to turn on a "skinny gene" when the body's healthy supply of energy is small by calories. However, there are few studies behind sort food. Research is still needed to understand Sirtuin and its effect on our healthfully.

Keto Diet: What Can You Eat

And now that part you were all waiting for ... what you can eat! A keto diet consists of lots of high-fat foods, which are probably already in your fridge.

Seafood

All vitamin-rich and keto-friendly, including Salmon, shrimp, halibut ... Be careful about specific types of shellfish, including palms, mustards, potatoes, and oysters, as high in carbs.

Low-carb vegetables

Eat enough, greens! Such as Brussels, broccoli, and asparagus are nutrient-dense veggies that the ketogenic diet can eat in abundance. The list continues. However, it's a keto-friendly veggie as far it has a low-carbohydrate count.

Cheese

Some of you say, Hallelujah! Yes, because it contains high-fat content, cheese is allowed in the keto diet. The best options are the mozzarella and cheddar cheeses. Be mindful of processed cheese and other high-sugar dairy products.

Avocados

The California "delicacy" is a thing to enjoy on the keto diet. Avocado is high in fatty acids and omega 3. Great when mixed with some vegetables in a smoothie or a meal and equally great as a snack.

Poultry and Meat

This is a staple of the keto diet. It has zero sugars and is full of useful vitamins. Suitable for meats higher in fat, like ribeye steaks and chicken thighs.

Eggs

Another great source of protein, omega-3-fatty acids, and essential nutrients are eggs to be eaten at breakfast or midday snacks.

Coconut oil

If you don't learn, cocoa oil is an excellent substitute for other cooking oils because when burnt at these high temperatures, it is safer. You know, it's suitable for rubbing on sunburn as you bounce on the beach showing your new bikini body from the keto diet.

Greek Yogurt

Another tasty choice, Greek yogurt for you to enjoy. It's nearly a dessert! Treat yourself! Treat yourself!

Cottage cheese

Not only a way to get your fats in, but it also helps to lower inflammation and heal muscles.

Sirtfood Diet: What Should You Eat?

Now that the long list of tasty things you will appreciate on the keto-diet is satisfied (and probably surprised), let's find out exactly what this mysterious "Sirtfood" is going and do it so that we will equate the two diet strategies.

Green Tea

This is a critical component of a Sirtfood diet, and green tea consists of an essential bioactive Sirtuin called catechin, which decreases oxidative stress and accelerates metabolism. This acts as an appetite suppressant and picks me up beautifully. The better you do!

Medjool Dates

Encouraged on diets of Sirtfood, Medjool dates are different from other periods because of the taste and texture they look like caramels.

They have lots of health advantages, and they are trendy during this diet. They go well in the smoothie, and they are also better eaten as snacks to please your mouth.

They also give excellent alternative tea or coffee sweetener.

Chocolate (must contain cocoa of at least 85%)

To eat a small quantity of dark chocolate in the Sirtfood Diet without thinking about it! Only make sure that the cocoa content is at least 85% or higher.

Apples

I know what they say. You know what they say. Eating an apple a day holds the doctor away, and an apple a day helps to prevent weight gain.

Tropical Fruits

And we realize that citrus fruit is low in minerals, antioxidants, and carbohydrates, but now we learn that it is abundant in polyphenol and that it allows our bodies to lose fat and lean.

Parsley

There are tons of antioxidants and minerals in this minty leaf. It supports bone safety and protects your view. To include the nutritional advantages of parsley as a garnish or blend with other cooked vegetables.

Turmeric

This is a welcome additive to this diet plan for a medicinal herb with anti-inflammatory effects. A dose of 500 to 2,000 milligrams- turmeric per day is healthy.

Kale

Among the world's most rich nutrient crops, kale can be eaten abundantly on the Sirtfood diet. Discover it in a smoothie or as a salad.

Berries

Blueberries are a delightful pleasure to indulge in this diet, Earth's flavor. They are also excellent for hydration and full of vitamins.

Capers

I bet that you did not realize the capers are an incredibly useful superfood. Caper can be used for diabetes, fungal infections, arthritis, and other conditions.

Red Wine

Furthermore, red wine with open arms is accepted on a Sirtfood diet (in moderation, of course). They aren't the only recipes you should appreciate. Others include coffee, arugula, chilies, walnuts, etc. But you get the spit!

Keto Diet Benefits vs. Sirtfood Diet Benefits

The two conventional diets tend to encourage you to consume a wide variety of items that you need to cut out with specific foods to reduce your lose. They deliver a much more practical and enjoyable menu than a claim, the diet for cod soup. The main problem now is: which is one of these two diets is better for you?

A Keto diet can assist you in losing weight and also boost your health. You will help to understand acne and increase the heart and brain's efficiency and reduce the chance of life-threatening illnesses, such as some cancers. This was also reported to help minimize convulsions of small children.

Studies have shown that you can adhere to your diet primarily with a ketogenic diet for the long term, but your wellbeing must add more carbs, such as vegetables, fruit, and beans.

On the other side, a Sirtfood diet was also selected as a means of quick weight loss. It can defend you from chronic diseases and has anti-aging capabilities. Whether or not you're rigid with this diet plan, including these nutrient - rich Sirt foods menu in your diet will improve your wellbeing.

Nonetheless, for several reasons, this lifestyle is not practical in the long term. The ultra-low-carb diet and low calorie may be dangerous, and more work is needed to determine the effect on our bodies.

Conclusively, it seems that the Keto diet and the Sirtfood diet have both positive and negative effects. The reality is that all significant dietary improvements are likely to help you shed weight, and these current, innovative plans are realistic choices when appropriately implemented.

The ultimate focus is both the keto and Sirtfood diets on nutrient-rich foods and the positive response in our bodies to a higher metabolism, reduced inflammation, and excess fat burning. Perhaps a combination of these two diets is the best of all worlds? We'll leave it to learn with some wellness authority.

If you have your own weight loss goals and want to try a new approach, lifestyle changes like the ketogenic or Sirt food diet are worth a shot. Some diet that makes dark chocolate, wine, or high-fat mozzarella cheese cannot be too challenging at the end of the day.

Chapter 4
What to Eat?

Sirtfoods are plant-based foods that activate a called a sirtuin. Sirtuins belong to a family of proteins that help insulate and protect our cells from damage, reducing our risk of developing any or all major diseases.

Many people turn to diets as a means of losing weight, and the Sirtfood Diet has been proven to be very good at helping achieve this goal. However, the interesting finding is that the diet isn't a weight management tool, so much as a strategy for enhancing overall health, in order to live longer, healthier lives, free from diabetes, heart disease, and even dementia. It simply turns out that healthy body weight is a natural by-product of good health.

Unfortunately, the Standard American Diet SAD, also sometimes referred to as the Western Pattern Diet WPD, is notably lacking in sirtfoods.

I'll introduce you to a list of the Top 20 Sirtfoods, which are featured prominently. I've also included a supplementary list of an additional 10 fruits and 10 vegetables that are also very rich in sirtuin-activators and also common throughout these recipes.

This makes the recipes not only feel somewhat familiar and achievable, but by sticking to the top sirtfoods, it makes shopping convenient and easy. You'll get to know the ingredients quickly and develop your confidence for tweaking recipes and developing your own, unique versions.

Healthy, home cooked food should never be boring or distasteful, and they don't have to be difficult either. Plants have such an incredible array of flavors and aromas that you'll find your Sirtfood meals exciting and packed with just as much flavor as nutrition.

Top 20 Sirtfoods

In Alphabetical Order:

- Arugula Rocket
- Buckwheat
- Capers
- Celery
- Chili's
- Cocoa
- Coffee
- Extra Virgin Olive Oil
- Garlic
- Green Tea
- Kale
- Medjool Dates
- Parsley
- Red Endive

- Red Onions
- Red Wine
- Soy
- Strawberries
- Turmeric
- Walnuts

Additional Sirtuin Rich Foods

Fruits

- Apples
- Blackberries
- Black currents
- Blueberries
- Citrus fruits
- Cranberries
- Goji berries
- Plums
- Raspberries
- Red Grapes

Vegetables and Herbs

- Artichokes
- Asparagus

- Broccoli

- Chia seeds

- Dill

- Green beans

- Lovage

- Quinoa

- Shallots

- Spinach

- Watercress

There are plenty of other vitamin rich and nutrient dense plants for you to add to your meals as well. Whenever you're in doubt or looking to experiment with new ingredients, simply look for the freshest, seasonal produce you can find, preferably in a wide array of colors. This combination will gift you with plenty of nutrition whether or not the individual items made the top 20 list of Sirtfoods.

As you're trying out the recipes on the following pages, don't be afraid to add or swap ingredients, especially if you know you detest certain options and can't get enough of others.

This guide is meant to last you a lifetime, so mark up the pages and add your own personal flair as you test out new dishes and become more and more addicted to the health and vitality that comes from eating a diverse, nutritional diet.

Chapter 5
Sirtfood Science

Sirtuins & Muscle Mass

We have mentioned how sirtuins help the body retain muscle mass even when dieting. How do this work? Well, sirtuins are a group of proteins with different effects.

Sirt-1 is the protein responsible for causing the body to burn fat rather than muscle for energy, which is obviously a miracle for weight loss. Another useful aspect of Sirt-1 is its ability to improve skeletal muscle.

Skeletal muscle is all the muscles you voluntarily control, such as the muscles in your limbs, back, shoulders and so on. There are two other types, cardiac muscle is what the heart is formed of, whilst smooth muscle is your involuntary muscles – which includes muscles around your blood vessels, face and various parts of organs and other tissues.

Skeletal muscle is separated into two different groups, the blandly named type-1 and type-2. Type 1 muscle is effective at continued, sustained activity whereas type-2 muscle is effective at short, intense periods of activity. So, for example, you would predominantly use type-1 muscles for jogging, but type-2 muscles for sprinting.

Sirt-1 protects the type-1 muscles, but not the type-2 muscle, which is still broken down for energy. Therefore, holistic muscle mass drops when fasting, even though type-1 skeletal muscle mass increases.

Sirt-1 also influences how the muscles actually work. Sirt-1 is produced by the muscle cells, but the ability to produce Sirt-1 decreases as the muscle ages. As a result, muscle is harder to build as you age and doesn't grow as fast in response to exercise. A lack of sirt-1 also causes the muscles to become tired quicker and gradually decline over time.

When you start to consider these effects of Sirt-1, you can start to form a picture about why fasting helps keep the body supple. Fasting releases Sirt-1, which in turn helps skeletal muscle grow and stay in good shape. Sirt-1 is also released by consuming sirtuin activators, giving the Sirtfood diet its muscle retaining power.

Sirtuins & Disease

The authors of the Sirtfood diet don't just claim that sirtuins can help improve skeletal muscle retention during dieting, but rather that they positively impact almost every dietary based disease in existence.

For example, one claim is that sirtuins help improve overall heart health by protecting and strengthening the cardiac.

Another claim expounded is that the Sirtfood diet also helps control diabetes. Some studies have found an association between Sirt-1 and the volume of insulin that can be released into the body. If you are familiar with the science behind diabetes, you may be aware that insulin is the hormone primarily responsible for controlling the levels of sugar in the blood. Therefore by increasing the amount of insulin that can be released, sirt-1 can theoretically help tackle diabetes by causing higher amounts of blood sugar to be converted into fat.

On top of this, sirtuins have been argued to influence Alzheimer's. Individuals with Alzheimer's have been found to have notably lower levels of sirtuins than healthy peers, although the mechanism of action between sirtuin and the disease is not fully understood.

The authors of the Sirtfood diet claims that sirtuins help prevent a build-up of the molecules amyloid-B and tau protein, which is responsible for the plaques that form in the brains of Alzheimer's sufferers and therefore all the corresponding symptoms. In fact, it isn't just argued that sirtuins help Alzheimer's, but also improves overall brain and cognitive function in regular people.

To add to the list of purported benefits is that sirtuins also help protect our bones. In particular, the specific argument is that sirtuin activation protects and helps retain our precious osteoblasts, which are a cell in our bones that allows more bone cells to be produced.

Finally, sirtuins have also been claimed to be a generic fighter against cancer, as they have supposedly have tumor suppression properties.

With all these claims, it is hard to discern fact from fiction. It does seem likely that a diet high in sirtuins does indeed have some of these benefits, but typically a diet high in sirtuins is more nutritious than an average Western diet. Therefore it is not yet determined whether sirtuins are the active component producing these effects, or different molecules also present in sirtfoods are responsible.

Sirtuins & Fat

Biology is far from straight-forward. You don't only have more than one type of muscle – you have more than one type of fat too. For our purposes, we are only going to focus on white adipose tissue and brown adipose tissue – two fancy terms for different kinds of fat.

White adipose tissue, or WAT as it is commonly abbreviated, is the fat made for storage. It's where your spare energy goes and having more WAT makes it easier to store and gain fat in future. Brown adipose tissue, or BAT, is a type of fat tissue that is typically associated with burning fat. BAT helps keeps us warm and contains high levels of mitochondria – the portion of the cell that is responsible for producing energy.

Leaner people actually have higher levels of brown fat than their overweight peers. BAT is located around the neck and back, whilst your WAT is located in the areas typically associated with obesity – your gut, buttocks, chest, hips. By having higher levels of BAT, fitter people have more ability to shake off calories through exercise and thermal release, so although research on BAT is still in its nascent stages, higher BAT levels and activity is hypothesized to be a good thing.

Of course, as you might now anticipate, sirtuins also affect our WAT and BAT levels. More precisely, sirtuins help convert your WAT into BAT, changing your body and making it easier to burn calories and lose weight. Over time this will produce large differences in your body composition, helping to not only make you lose weight, but become lean and fit.

Sirtfoods & Your Diet

By now, we have talked about how sirtuins are proteins produced by genes in our body, which demonstrate numerous beneficial effects on the body. We all have noted three primary means of causing sirtuins to be released in the body; eating to a calorie deficit, stringent fasting and exercise.

One of the primary claims of the Sirtfood diet is that sirtuins can also be released through your diet, with the most potent sirtuin-releasing foods nicknamed Sirtfoods. Let us examine this claim in more detail.

It is known that a nutritionally rich diet, especially a diet high in fruit and vegetables, drastically reduces the risk of cancer and a legion of diseases. The reason why this is true has been attributed to many different factors, such as the increasingly popular 'anti-oxidants' as well as higher levels of mineral and vitamins in these foods.

Yet this isn't the rationale of why the Sirtfood diet advocates so many plants and vegetables. Instead the argument rests upon Sirtfoods being special, above and beyond all other components of our food. This argument actually rests upon the toxic qualities of the Sirtfoods, rather than their nutritional superiority.

Now, this is perhaps the most fascinating aspect of the Sirtfood diet. The two authors of this diet argue that all the things we associate with improving our health exercise, fasting, and calorie restriction all have a minor stress component. Essentially these activities put the body into a minor state of stress, causing the body to enact processes that help us adapt and improve.

This concept is called hormesis and is basically the idea of what doesn't kill you, makes you stronger. Or in more scientific terms, small doses of certain harmful substances can produce a positive effect via the triggering of biological adaptations.

Plants themselves can have hormesis reactions to stressors in their environment. In fact, plant hormesis is rather sophisticated and plants, being stationary, have much more nuanced and varied stress reactions than mammals and humans.

To bring it all together, eating these hormones and chemicals from 'stressed' plants can also benefit us, as some of our biological adaptations involve usage of the same chemicals and hormones. In particular, polyphenols are known to benefit the human body and trigger sirtuin release.

This concept, of using plants stress-reactions to benefit our own is a field of study called xenohormesis. This is the very basis of Sirtfoods; sirtfoods are good for us because they contain sirtuins, which are molecules released in stress-reactions in plants, which also help our body adapt and improve.

How Much Sirtfood's Do You Need To Eat?

Of course, the Sirtfood diet is more than just pumping a bunch of the best Sirtfoods into your eating habits. It is a holistic diet with food organized into different meals, each designed to give you the highest sirtuin kick. On top of this, the Sirtfood diet isn't exotic.

The main ingredients of the Sirtfood diet are common and you probably use them already, on occasion. The trick is just making sure you are getting enough – the average American only receives 13mg of sirtuins a day – which is five times lower than their Japanese counterparts.

So if Sirtuins are so fantastic, why don't we take them as a supplement or pill? The truth is although a pharmaceutical application of sirtuins may be possible in the future our current understanding of food science and biology is still too limited for this to be effective today.

Understanding how sirtuins are processed and absorbed, which likely depends on other nutrients in food, is crucial to making sirtuins actually work. At the moment, it is simply easier and more successful to consume sirtuins the natural way, receiving all the extra stuff you need in the sirtfoods themselves.

For example, resveratrol, the sirtuin activator which is present in certain types of red wine, is known to be absorbed poorly when taken are a pure substance. When ingested in red-wine, it is in fact absorbed six times better. Simply put, food is complicated and we only understand a few pieces of the puzzle.

Another reason why sirtuins are not taken as a pill or supplement is the fact there are so many of them, all with slightly different effects. Add this to the before mentioned complexity and its better just to consume foods where you know you get a natural mix.

Fighting Fats through Sirtuins

Ecological factors significantly influence the destiny of living beings and sustenance is one of the most persuasive variables. These days life span is a significant objective of medicinal science and has consistently been a fabrication for the individual since antiquated occasions. Specifically, endeavors are planned for accomplishing effective maturing, to be specific a long life without genuine ailments, with a decent degree of physical and mental autonomy and satisfactory social connections.

Gathering information unmistakably exhibits that it is conceivable to impact the indications of maturing. Without a doubt, wholesome mediations can advance wellbeing and life span. It is commonly valued that the sort of diet can significantly impact the quality and amount of life and the Mediterranean eating regimen is paradigmatic of an advantageous dietary example

Chapter 6
Breakfast Recipes

1. Omelet with Peppers

Preparation Time: 10 minutes

Cooking Time: 15 minutes

Servings: 4

Ingredients

4 eggs, beaten
1 tablespoon margarine

1 cup bell peppers, chopped
2 oz scallions, chopped

Directions

Toss the margarine in the skillet and melt it.
In the mixing bowl mix up eggs and bell peppers. Add scallions.
Pour the egg mixture in the hot skillet and roast the omelet for 12 minutes.

Nutrition

Calories: 102
Protein: 6.1g
Sugar: 3g
Fiber: 0.8g

Carbohydrates: 7.3g
Fat: 10.8g
Sodium: 98mg

2. Quinoa Hashes

Preparation Time: 10 minutes

Cooking Time: 25inutes

Servings: 2

Ingredients

3 oz quinoa

2 potatoes, grated

1 tablespoon avocado oil

6 oz water

1 egg, beaten

1 teaspoon chives, chopped

Directions

Cook quinoa in water for 15 minutes.

Heat up avocado oil in the skillet.

Then mix up all remaining ingredients in the bowl. Add quinoa and mix up well.

Add quinoa hash browns, cook for 5 minutes on each side.

Nutrition

Calories: 344

Protein: 12.5.g

Sugar: 0.2g

Fiber: 3.4g

Carbohydrates: 5.9g

Fat: 5.9g

Sodium: 388mg

3. Artichoke Eggs

Preparation Time: 5 minutes

Cooking Time: 20 minutes

Servings: 4

Ingredients ·

5 eggs, beaten
1 yellow onion, chopped
1 tablespoon cilantro, chopped
1 cup artichoke hearts, canned, chopped

2 oz low-fat feta, chopped
1 tablespoon canola oil

Directions ·

Grease 4 ramekins with the oil.
Mix up all remaining ingredients and divide the mixture between prepared ramekins.
Bake the meal at 380F for 20 minutes.

Nutrition ·

Calories: 177
Protein: 10.6g
Sugar: 1g
Fiber: 2g

Carbohydrates: 7.4g
Fat: 12.2g
Sodium: 259mg

4. Quinoa Cakes

Preparation Time: 10 minutes

Cooking Time: 25 minutes

Servings: 4

Ingredients

7 oz quinoa
1 cup of water
1 egg, beaten
½ teaspoon ground black pepper

1 cup cauliflower, shredded
½ cup vegan parmesan, grated
1 tablespoon olive oil

Directions

Mix up the quinoa with the cauliflower, water, and ground black pepper, stir, bring to a simmer over medium heat and cook for 15 minutes.

Cool the mixture and add parmesan and the eggs, stir well, shape medium cakes out of this mix.

Heat up a pan with the oil over medium-high heat, add the quinoa cakes. Cook them for 4-5 minutes per side.

Nutrition

Calories: 280
Protein: 25.4g
Sugar: 1.2g
Fiber: 1g

Carbohydrates: 6.8g
Fat: 7.6g
Sodium: 222mg

5. Bean Casserole

Preparation Time: 10 minutes

Cooking Time: 30 minutes

Servings: 8

Ingredients

5 eggs, beaten   ½ cup bell pepper, chopped
1 cup beans, cooked   ½ cup onions, chopped
1 cup low-fat mozzarella cheese, shredded

Directions

Spread the beans over the casserole mold. Add onions and bell pepper.
Add the eggs mixed with the cheese.
Bake the casserole 380 F for 30 minutes.

Nutrition

Calories: 142   Carbohydrates: 16g
Protein: 23.8g   Fat: 3g
Sugar: 0.2g   Sodium: 162mg
Fiber: 2.3g

6. Blueberry Muffins

Preparation Time: 15 minutes

Cooking Time: 20 minutes

Servings: 8

Ingredients

1 cup buckwheat flour   ¼ cup arrowroot starch
1½ teaspoons baking powder   ¼ teaspoon sea salt
2 eggs   ½ cup almond milk
2–3 tablespoons maple syrup   1 cup fresh blueberries
2 tablespoons coconut oil, melted

Directions

Preheat your oven to 350ºF and line 8 cups of a muffin tin. In a bowl, place the buckwheat flour, arrowroot starch, baking powder, and salt, and mix well.
In a separate bowl, place the eggs, almond milk, maple syrup, and coconut oil, and beat until well combined.
Now, place the flour mixture and mix until just combined. Gently, fold in the blueberries. Transfer the mixture into prepared muffin cups evenly. Bake for about 25 minutes or until a toothpick inserted in the center comes out clean.
Remove the muffin tin from oven and place onto a wire rack to cool for about 10 minutes. Carefully invert the muffins onto the wire rack to cool completely before serving.

Nutrition

Calories 136   Fat 5.3 g
Carbs 20.7 g   Protein 3.5 g

7. Salmon & Kale Omelet

Preparation Time: 10 minutes

Cooking Time: 7 minutes

Servings: 4

Ingredients
6 eggs

2 tablespoons almond milk

2 tablespoons olive oil

Salt and ground black pepper

4 ounces smoked salmon, cut into bite-sized chunks

2 cup fresh kale, tough ribs removed and chopped finely

4 scallions, chopped finely

Directions

In a bowl, place the eggs, coconut milk, salt, and black pepper, and beat well. Set aside.

In a non-stick wok, heat the oil over medium heat.

Place the egg mixture evenly and cook for about 30 seconds, without stirring.

Place the salmon kale and scallions on top of egg mixture evenly.

Now, reduce heat to low.

With the lid, cover the wok and cook for about 4–5 minutes, or until omelet is done completely.

Uncover the wok and cook for about 1 minute.

Carefully, transfer the omelet onto a serving plate and serve.

Nutrition

Calories 210

Fat 14.9 g

Carbs 5.2 g

Protein 14.8 g

8. Moroccan Spiced Eggs

Preparation Time: 1 hour

Cooking Time: 50 minutes

Servings: 2

Ingredients

1 tsp olive oil

½ tsp gentle stew powder

¼ tsp ground cinnamon

4 eggs at room temperature

1 tbsp tomato puree (glue)

¼ tsp ground cumin

½ tsp salt

1 shallot, stripped and hacked

1 red (chime) pepper, deseeded and hacked

1 garlic clove, stripped and hacked

1 corvette (zucchini), stripped and hacked

1 × 400g (14oz) can hacked tomatoes

1 x 400g (14oz) may chickpeas in water

10g (1/3 oz) level leaf parsley, cleaved

Directions

Heat the oil in a pan, include the shallot and red (ringer) pepper and fry delicately for 5 minutes. At that point include the garlic and courgette (zucchini) and cook for one more moment or two. Include the tomato puree (glue), flavors and salt and mix through.

Add the cleaved tomatoes and chickpeas (dousing alcohol and all) and increment the warmth to medium. With the top of the dish, stew the sauce for 30 minutes – ensure it is delicately rising all through and permit it to lessen in volume by around 33%.

Remove from the warmth and mix in the cleaved parsley.

Preheat the grill to 200C/180C fan/350F.

When you are prepared to cook the eggs, bring the tomato sauce up to a delicate stew and move to a little broiler confirmation dish.

Crack the eggs on the dish and lower them delicately into the stew. Spread with thwart and prepare in the grill for 10-15 minutes. Serve the blend in unique dishes with the eggs coasting on the top.

Nutrition

Calories: 116 kcal

Fat: 5.22 g

Protein: 6.97 g

Carbohydrates: 13.14 g

9. Chilaquiles with Gochujang

Preparation Time: 30 minutes

Cooking Time: 20 minutes

Servings: 2

Ingredients

One dried ancho Chile
2 cups of water
1 cup squashed tomatoes
Two cloves of garlic
One teaspoon genuine salt
1/2 tablespoons gochujang
5 to 6 cups tortilla chips
Three enormous eggs
One tablespoon olive oil

Directions

Get the water to heat a pot. I cheated marginally and heated the water in an electric pot and emptied it into the pan. There's no sound unrivalled strategy here. Add the anchor Chile to the bubbled water and drench for 15 minutes to give it an opportunity to stout up.

When completed, use tongs or a spoon to extricate Chile. Make sure to spare the water for the sauce! Nonetheless, on the off chance that you incidentally dump the water, it's not the apocalypse.

Mix the doused Chile, 1 cup of saved high temp water, squashed tomatoes, garlic, salt and gochujang until smooth. Empty sauce into a large dish and warmth over medium warmth for 4 to 5 minutes. Mood killer the heat and include the tortilla chips. Mix the chips to cover with the sauce. In a different skillet, shower a teaspoon of oil and fry an egg on top, until the whites have settled. Plate the egg and cook the remainder of the eggs. If you are phenomenal at performing various tasks, you can likely sear the eggs while you heat the red sauce. I am not precisely so capable.

Top the chips with the seared eggs, cotija, hacked cilantro, jalapeños, onions and avocado. Serve right away.

Nutrition

Calories: 484 kcal

Fat: 18.62 g

Protein: 14.55 g

Carbohydrates: 64.04 g

10. Sirtfood Baked Breakfast Potatoes

Preparation Time: 1 hour 10 minutes

Cooking Time: 1 hour

Servings: 2

Ingredients ·

2 tablespoons unsalted spread   4 rashers cooked bacon
4 huge eggs   ½ cup destroyed cheddar
Daintily cut chives   Salt and pepper to taste
3 tablespoons overwhelming cream
2 medium reddish-brown potatoes, cleaned and pricked with a fork everywhere

Directions ·

Preheat grill to 400°F.

Spot potatoes straightforwardly on stove rack in the focal point of the grill and prepare for 30 to 45 min.

Evacuate and permit potatoes to cool for around 15 minutes.

Cut every potato down the middle longwise and burrow every half out, scooping the potato substance into a blending bowl.

Gather margarine and cream to the potato and pound into a single unit until smooth — season with salt and pepper and mix.

Spread a portion of the potato blend into the base of each emptied potato skin and sprinkle with one tablespoon cheddar (you may make them remain pounded potato left to snack on).

Add one rasher bacon to every half and top with a raw egg.

Spot potatoes onto a heating sheet and come back to the

appliance.

Lower broiler temperature to 375°F and heat potatoes until egg whites simply set and yolks are as yet runny.

Top every potato with a sprinkle of the rest of the cheddar, season with salt and pepper and finish with cut chives.

Nutrition ·

Calories: 647 kcal

Fat: 55.79 g

Protein: 30.46 g

Carbohydrates: 7.45 g

Chapter 7
Juice Recipes

11. Banana Juice Shake With Cream

Preparation Time: 5 minutes

Cooking Time: 0 minutes

Servings: 2

Ingredients

3 bananas, peeled
6 ice cubes, divided
3 mango slices, cut into cubes

1 cup water
1 cup whipped cream

Directions

In a blender, blend mango and bananas for 2 minutes until smooth. Put in 3 ice cubes and process for 2 minutes, until smooth. Fill the leftover 3 ice cubes into a cocktail shaker, then put in blended banana mixture.

Cover and shake until the outside of shaker has frosted. Strain into 2 cold glasses and decorate with whipped cream.

Nutrition

Calories: 381
Protein: 4.6g
Sugar: 1.5g
Fiber: 2.3g

Carbohydrates: 82.1g
Fat: 2g
Sodium: 51mg

12. Turmeric Ginger C Boost Life Juice

Preparation Time: 5 minutes

Cooking Time: 0 minutes

Servings: 1

Ingredients

1/2 tsp. ground turmeric   2 Fuji apples, cored and sliced
1/2 lemon, peeled   1 (1 inch) piece fresh ginger
1 orange, peeled and divided

Directions

With a juicer, process ginger, lemon, orange and apples, then stir in turmeric until evenly combined.

Nutrition

Calories: 163   Carbohydrates: 45.6 g
Protein: 3 g   Fat: 0.6g
Sugar: 1g   Sodium: 87mg
Fiber: 0.7 g

13. V-great Juice

Preparation Time: 15 minutes

Cooking Time: 0 minutes

Servings: 1

Ingredients

4 tomatoes
4 stalks celery
3 radishes
1/4 lemon, peeled
1/2 cup mixed spring greens, or to taste

4 carrots
2 leaves kale
1/4 lemon, with rind

Directions

Run lemon, radishes, kale, spring greens, celery, carrots and tomatoes with rind, then peeled lemon through a juicer following the manufacturer's instructions.

Nutrition

Calories: 288
Protein: 6g
Sugar: 1.3g
Fiber: 4g

Carbohydrates: 43.6 g
Fat: 0.8g
Sodium: 98mg

14. Ginger-beet Juice

Preparation Time: 15 minutes

Cooking Time: 0 minutes

Servings: 2

Ingredients

1 orange, peeled and quartered
1 apple, cut into wedges
1 inch piece peeled fresh ginger
1 large beet, peeled and cut into wedges

3 kale leaves
1 carrot, peeled
Ice cubes (optional)

Directions

Following the manufacturer's instructions to process through a juicer with orange, kale, apple, carrot, beet and ginger, respectively in this order.
Fill 2 glasses with ice, if wanted, and pour the juice into the glasses.
Serve promptly.

Nutrition

Calories: 223
Protein: 1.8g
Sugar: 2.5g
Fiber: 0g

Carbohydrates: 21g
Fat: 2g
Sodium: 56mg

15. Heavenly Honeydew Juice

Preparation Time: 10 minutes

Cooking Time: 0 minutes

Servings: 6

Ingredients

2 cups ice cubes   1 cup water
3 tbsps. White sugar
1 (5 lb.) honeydew melon, quartered and seeded

Directions

Scrape into a blender with the meat from honeydew melon quarters, then put into the blender with sugar, water and ice cubes.
Process until smooth and sugar is dissolved and serve promptly.

Nutrition

Calories: 259   Carbohydrates: 40.3g
Protein: 2g   Fat: 2g
Sugar: 2.5g   Sodium: 76mg
Fiber: 0.3g

16. Orange-Carrot-Ginger Juice

Preparation Time: 15 minutes

Cooking Time: 0 minutes

Servings: 1

Ingredients ·

1 large orange, peeled
1/4 cup lemon juice
Ice

1 cup carrots, chopped
1 (1 inch) piece ginger

Directions ·

In a juicer, add ginger, lemon juice, carrots and orange, then following the manufacturer's instruction to blend until smooth.
Transfer the juice into a glass filled with ice.

Nutrition ·

Calories: 150
Protein: 1g
Sugar: 1g
Fiber: 0g

Carbohydrates: 34g
Fat: 0.3g
Sodium: 93mg

17. Hot Caramel Apple Juice

Preparation Time: 5 minutes

Cooking Time: 0 minutes

Servings: 2

Ingredients

2 cups apple juice
1 tsp. ground cinnamon
1/4 tsp. vanilla extract
1/4 cup whipped cream, or to taste (optional)

3 tbsps. Caramel syrup
1/2 tsp. ground nutmeg

Directions

In a saucepan, whisk together nutmeg, cinnamon, caramel syrup and apple juice on medium high heat.
Cook and whisk briskly for 3 minutes, until the mixture is hot without boiling.
Put in vanilla, then cook and stir for 1 minute longer.
Transfer into the mugs and place whipped cream on top.

Nutrition

Calories: 222
Protein: 1g
Sugar: 0.2g
Fiber: 0g

Carbohydrates: 34g
Fat: 0.5g
Sodium: 64mg

18. Delicious Green Juice

Preparation Time: 5 minutes

Cooking Time: 0 minutes

Servings: 1

Ingredients

1 cup coconut milk   3/4 cup fresh spinach, or to taste
1 banana   1 mango - peeled, seeded, and chopped

Directions

Blend the banana, spinach, coconut milk, and mango in the blender until it is smooth.

Nutrition

Calories: 191   Carbohydrates: 48g
Protein: 3g   Fat: 1g
Sugar: 1g   Sodium: 89mg
Fiber: 1g

19. Fresh, Homemade Apple Juice

Preparation Time: 10 minutes

Cooking Time: 0 minutes

Servings: 5

Ingredients

5 cups water   1/4 cup white sugar
3 peels and cores from red apples - seeds removed

Directions

Put into saucepan with cores and peelings, then stir in the water. Bring the mixture to a boil, then lower heat to a simmer and cook for a half hour while stirring sometimes, until the water picks up the apple flavor and color.
Drain apple juice and get rid of the solid pieces, then stir in the sugar until dissolved.
Let juice cool before drink.

Nutrition

Calories: 388   Carbohydrates: 32g
Protein: 1g   Fat: 0.5g
Sugar: 0.8g   Sodium: 63mg
Fiber: 1g

Chapter 8
Smoothie Recipes

20. Creamy Mango Smoothie

Preparation Time: 5 minutes

Cooking Time: 0 minutes

Servings: 2

Ingredients

3/4 cup cold milk   1/4 cup vanilla yogurt
3/4 tsp. vanilla extract   3 ice cubes
1 1/2 cups chopped fresh mango

Directions

Using a blender, blend together ice cubes, mango, vanilla extract, yogurt, and milk until it is all creamy and smooth.

Nutrition

Calories: 154   Carbohydrates: 29.8g
Protein: 2g   Fat: 1g
Sugar: 0.5g   Sodium: 98mg;
Fiber: 1g

21. Easy Mango Banana Smoothie

Preparation Time: 10 minutes

Cooking Time: 0 minutes

Servings: 1

Ingredients

2 mangos - peeled, seeded, and sliced   2 bananas
2 cups vanilla yogurt   2 cups milk

Directions

In a blender, conflate milk, vanilla yogurt, banana and mangos till smooth.

Nutrition

Calories: 133   Carbohydrates: 34g
Protein: 3g   Fat: 1g
Sugar: 2g   Sodium: 72mg
Fiber: 0g

22. Easy Mango Lassi

Preparation Time: 10 minutes

Cooking Time: 0 minutes

Servings: 4

Ingredients ·

2 cups plain whole milk yogurt   1 cup milk
1/8 tsp. ground cardamom   4 tsps. White sugar
3 mangoes - peeled, seeded, and chopped

Directions ·

In the jar of a blender, place cardamom, white sugar, mangoes, milk, and yogurt.
Blend together for about 2 minutes or until smooth.
Chill in the refrigerator until cold, about 1 hour.
Serve with a bit sprinkling of ground cardamom.

Nutrition ·

Calories: 184   Carbohydrates: 48g
Protein: 0.8g   Fat: 1.8g
Sugar 0.6g   Sodium: 64mg
Fiber: 0.5g

23. Gloomy Day Smoothie

Preparation Time: 10 minutes

Cooking Time: 0 minutes

Servings: 4

Ingredients

1 banana, peeled and chopped   1 cup orange juice
1 cup vanilla nonfat yogurt
1 mango - peeled, seeded, and cut into chunks

Directions

Put the banana, mango, orange juice, and yogurt in a blender and blend until the mix is smooth.
Fill up clear glasses, add a bendy straw for drinking and serve!

Nutrition

Calories: 203
Protein: 1.2g
Sugar: 2g
Fiber: 1g

Carbohydrates: 34g
Fat: 2g
Sodium: 83mg

24. Happy Skinny Green Smoothie

Preparation Time: 10 minutes

Cooking Time: 0 minutes

Servings: 1

Ingredients

2 green tea bags
1/2 lime, juiced
1 cup fresh mango chunks
1/2 avocado, peeled and pitted
1/2 cup green seedless grapes
2 cups loosely packed organic baby spinach
1/4 cup loosely packed fresh mint leaves
1 (1/2- by 1/4-inch) piece fresh ginger, chopped

1 1/2 cups boiling water
1/2 green apple, chopped
2 packets Organic Stevia

Directions

Get boiling water and soak the tea bags in it for 3-5 minutes.
Remove the tea bags and allow the tea to cool.
Once cooled, pour it into the blender together with the rest
of the ingredients and process until it is smooth.
Serve right away.

Nutrition

Calories: 222
Protein: 8g
Sugar: 2g
Fiber: 0g

Carbohydrates: 59.3g
Fat: 1.6g
Sodium: 59mg

25. Holly Goodness Smoothie

Preparation Time: 10 minutes

Cooking Time: 0 minutes

Servings: 1

Ingredients

1 small banana
1/2 cup almond milk
1 tsp. vanilla extract
1 tsp. hemp seeds
1 mango - peeled, seeded, and chopped

1/2 cup frozen raspberries
1/2 cup hemp milk
1 tsp. chia seeds
1 tsp. maca powder

Directions

Blend together maca powder, hemp seeds, chia seeds, vanilla extract, hemp milk, almond milk, raspberries, banana, and mango using a blender until the mixture is smooth.

Nutrition

Calories: 383
Protein: 3g
Sugar: 1.3g
Fiber: 0g

Carbohydrates: 76g
Fat: 1g
Sodium: 63mg

26. Honey-mango Smoothie

Preparation Time: 10 minutes

Cooking Time: 0 minutes

Servings: 2

Ingredients •

1 tbsp. white sugar   2 tbsps. Honey
1 cup nonfat milk   1 tsp. lemon juice
1 cup ice cubes   1 mango - peeled, seeded, and cubed

Directions •

In a blender pitcher, put sugar, honey and mango; add lemon juice and milk, conflate till smooth. Distribute ice cubes among 2 serving glasses.
Put mango smoothie on ice, serve.

Nutrition •

Calories: 346   Carbohydrates: 45g
Protein: 1.8g   Fat: 2g
Sugar: 0.5g   Sodium: 58mg
Fiber: 0.4g

27. Hong Kong Mango Drink

Preparation Time: 10 minutes

Cooking Time: 0 minutes

Servings: 2

Ingredients

1/2 cup small pearl tapioca
1 mango - peeled, seeded and diced
14 ice cubes
1/2 cup coconut milk

Directions

Over high heat, boil water. When the water is boiling, mix in the tapioca pearls then boil again.

Uncover while cooking the tapioca pearls for 10 minutes, mixing from time to time. Put the cover back then take off heat, let it rest for half an hour.

In a colander placed in the sink, drain well; cover then chill. In a blender, blend ice and mango till smooth. In 2 tall glasses, distribute chilled tapioca pearls; pour the mango mixture on top then pour on top of each with a quarter cup coconut milk.

Nutrition

Calories: 234
Protein: 4.8g
Sugar: 3g
Fiber: 0g

Carbohydrates: 56g
Fat: 1g
Sodium: 64mg

28. Coconut-Blueberry Green Smoothie

Preparation Time: 5 minutes

Cooking Time: 0 minutes

Servings: 1

Ingredients

¾ cup frozen blueberries
¾ cup lightly packed baby spinach
1 cup unsweetened coconut milk beverage
½ cup low-fat plain Greek yogurt
1 tbsp. chia or hemp seeds
1 tbsp. maple syrup or agave nectar (optional)

Directions

Use a blender to mix the yogurt, blueberries, maple syrup (or agave) if available, spinach, coconut milk and chia (or hemp) together.
Let the blender run until the mixture is smooth in consistency, scrape the sides of the blender down 1 or 2 times to evenly blend the mixture.

Nutrition

Calories: 104
Protein: 2g
Sugar: 1g
Fiber: 1.2g

Carbohydrates: 24.1g
Fat: 0.4g
Sodium: 103mg

29. Mango Piña Colada Smoothie

Preparation Time: 5 minutes

Cooking Time: 0 minutes

Servings: 1

Ingredients

1 cup nonfat plain Greek yogurt
¾ cup frozen pineapple
¾ cup frozen mango
½ cup «lite» coconut milk (see Tip)
Unsweetened coconut flakes for garnish

Directions

Use a blender to mix the coconut milk, yogurt, pineapple and mango together.
Blend until the consistency is smooth. Top it with coconut flakes if you want.

Nutrition

Calories: 311
Protein: 2g
Sugar: 0g
Fiber: 1g

Carbohydrates: 49.6g
Fat: 0.4g
Sodium: 61mg

30. Jack-o'-lantern Smoothie Bowl

Preparation Time: 10 minutes

Cooking Time: 0 minutes

Servings: 1

Ingredients

1 cup frozen mango chunks
¾ cup reduced fat plain Greek yogurt
¼ cup reduced-fat milk
1 tsp. vanilla extract
1 strawberry, hulled and halved
1 tsp. chia seeds

Directions

In a blender, combine vanilla, milk, yogurt, and mango.
Puree the mixture until smooth.
Pour the entire smoothie into a bowl and decorate to make the drink look like a jack-o'-lantern.
Use halved strawberries to make the cheeks and use the chia seeds to make eyes and a nose.
Serve the smoothie with a green spoon attached with a paper leaf to make it look like a pumpkin stem.

Nutrition

Calories: 498
Protein: 1g
Sugar: 3g
Fiber: 1g

Carbohydrates: 56g
Fat: 1g
Sodium: 36mg

Chapter 9
Lunch Recipes

31. Cherry Chicken Lettuce Wraps

Preparation Time: 15 minutes

Cooking Time: 10 minutes

Servings: 1

Ingredients

12 lettuce leaves

2 tbsp rice vinegar

2 tbsp teriyaki sauce

1/2 cup green onion, diced

1 1/2 cups carrots, roughly cut

2 tbsp canola oil, separated

1/3 cup sliced almonds, toasted

1 tbsp honey

1 tbsp fresh ginger root, thinly cut

1 lb. dark sweet cherries, cut in halves and the pits removed

1 1/4 lb chicken breast, the skin and bones removed and minced

Directions

Set your stove to medium high heat and place a large sized skillet on it. Add 1 tbsp of oil to the pan and let it get hot. Put the skinless and boneless chicken in the pot and add your ginger. Sauté for 10 minutes. Be careful not to burn your chicken. You just want to make sure it is cooked through.

Get a bowl and add honey, vinegar, 1 tbsp oil, and teriyaki sauce. Using a whisk, mix these ingredients well, before throwing in your almonds, the chicken mixture in your skillet, green onion, cherries and carrots.

Using a spoon, place the mixture in the center of each of the twelve lettuce leaves. Roll the lettuce to cover this filling, and they are ready to serve.

Nutrition

Calories: 297
Protein: 25g
Sugar: 2g
Fiber: 1g

Carbohydrates: 21.5g
Fat: 12.4g
Sodium: 156mg

32. Easy Korean Beef

Preparation Time: 10 minutes

Cooking Time: 10 minutes

Servings: 4

Ingredients

1 tbsp sesame seeds
2 tbsp green onion, diced
2 cups cauliflower rice
¼ tsp ground black pepper
¼ tsp ground ginger

2 tsp sesame oil
1 lb. lean ground beef
3 garlic cloves, thinly cut
¼ cup soy sauce
1 tbsp coconut sugar

Directions

Make sure your stove is set to medium high heat and place a large skillet on it. Pour the sesame oil in the pan to make it hot, before adding garlic and ground beef.

After 7 minutes, by which time the beef would crumble easily, turn down the stove to low and quickly continue with the following step.

Grab a bowl and throw your black pepper, soy sauce, ginger, and coconut sugar in it. Using a whisk, mix these ingredients properly.

Now, you can pour the coconut sugar mixture over the cooked beef that is still in the pan. Increase the heat back to medium and let the beef mixture simmer for about 3 minutes.

Serve the keto Korean beef on top of your prepared cauliflower rice.

Finally, garnish with sesame seeds and green onions.

Nutrition ●

Calories: 297
Protein: 22.4g
Sugar: 0.6g
Fiber: 3.7g

Carbohydrates: 8.9g
Fat: 13.3g
Sodium: 956mg

33. Peanut Sesame Shirataki Noodles

Preparation Time: 20 minutes

Cooking Time: 10 minutes

Servings: 4

Ingredients

1 8 oz pack shirataki noodles
2 tbsp creamy peanut butter
1 medium carrot, shredded
1 tbsp soy sauce, low sodium
Toasted sesame seeds
Green onions
Cilantro
Pinch ground ginger

Snow peas
1 tbsp water
Peanuts
1 tsp rice vinegar
Pinch garlic powder
¼ tsp black pepper
1 tsp brown sugar
⅛ tsp sesame oil

Directions

Grab a medium sized bowl and put the ground ginger, peanut butter, sesame oil, water, brown sugar, soy sauce, black pepper, rice vinegar, and garlic powder inside it. Mix properly and set the bowl aside for 30 minutes.

Next, pop that bowl in the refrigerator until you have to use it on the pasta.

To prepare the pasta

Rinse your shirataki noodles. Follow that by draining the noodles and patting them dry using a paper towel.

Get a nonstick pan and place it over medium low heat. The pan has to be completely dry before the noodles. The purpose of this is to make further sure that the noodles are not wet. Do not burn them.

Chop your snow peas and add them, along with the grated carrots, into the pan containing your noodles. Sauté for about 4 minutes before you pour the sauce in. Mix the sauce into the other ingredients well.

Decorate with cilantro, toasted sesame seeds, green onions, and peanuts. Alternatively, you can choose not to garnish the meal.

Nutrition

Calories: 111
Protein: 12.6g
Sugar: 1.9g
Fiber: 2g

Carbohydrates: 9g
Fat: 6.5g
Sodium: 564mg

34. Ginger Asian Slaw

Preparation Time: 15 minutes

Cooking Time: 0 minutes

Servings: 8

Ingredients

Sea salt to your preferred taste
6 cups Napa cabbage, minced
Pepper to your preferred taste
6 cups red cabbage, minced
1 cup cilantro, shredded
¼ tsp cayenne pepper
¾ cup diced green onions
1 tbsp extra virgin olive oil
1 ½ inch ginger, shredded
1 tbsp apple cider vinegar
3 tbsp lime juice
2 cups carrots grated
1 medium lime zest
1 tbsp maple syrup
2 tbsp almond butter
1 tsp sesame oil
1 garlic clove, thinly cut
1 tbsp rice vinegar
2 tbsp tamari

Directions

Into the cup of a blender add your olive oil, salt, pepper, maple syrup, lime juice, sesame oil, lime zest, apple cider vinegar, cayenne pepper, tamari, garlic rice vinegar, ginger, and almond butter. Blend these ingredients until you are left with a smooth mixture. This is your dressing.

Next, you'll need a large mixing bowl. Put the cilantro, cabbage, green onions, and carrots inside it. Pour the mixture in your blender into the bowl and toss well.

For about an hour, let the bowl stay in your fridge. The various flavors will meld deliciously and afterwards, you can serve.

Nutrition •

Calories: 144
Protein: 24.4g
Sugar: 1.7g
Fiber: 1.7g

Carbohydrates: 12g
Fat: 6g
Sodium: 432mg

35. Zucchini Cream

Preparation Time: 10 minutes

Cooking Time: 25 minutes

Servings: 8

Ingredients

4 cups vegetable stock
8 zucchinis, chopped
1 cup coconut milk
1 teaspoon dried rosemary
4 tablespoons fresh dill, chopped
½ teaspoon fresh basil, chopped
2 sweet potatoes, peeled and cubed
2 tablespoons olive oil
2 onions, peeled and chopped
A pinch of salt and black pepper

Directions

Heat a pot with the oil over medium heat, add the onion, stir, and cook for 2 minutes. Add the zucchinis and the rest of the ingredients except the milk and dill, stir and simmer for 20 minutes.
Add the milk and dill, puree the soup using an immersion blender, stir, ladle into soup bowls and serve.

Nutrition

Calories: 324
Protein: 14.8g
Sugar: 1.8g
Fiber: 0.4g
Carbohydrates: 10g
Fat: 3g
Sodium: 585mg

36. Spicy Steak Rolls

Preparation Time: 20 minutes

Cooking Time: 1 hour 15 minutes

Servings: 4

Ingredients

10 slices bacon, chopped
1 green bell pepper, chopped
1 clove garlic, minced, or to taste
1/2 cup Montreal steak seasoning
1 (8 oz.) package fresh mushrooms, chopped

Toothpicks
1/2 small onion, chopped
4 beef round steaks

Directions

In a large skillet, sauté bacon for about 10 minutes over medium-high heat until evenly browned.

Add garlic, onion, green bell pepper, and mushrooms; sauté for about 10 minutes until mushrooms are tender. Put off the heat. Turn an outdoor grill to medium-high and lightly grease the grate.

On a flat work surface, position a round steak between 2 pieces of plastic wrap. Use a meat tenderizer to flatten the steak. Do the same with the remaining steaks.

Place Montreal steak seasoning into a shallow bowl. Dip 1 side of each steak into the seasoning and place on a cutting board, seasoning-side down. Spread some of the mushroom mixture over the center of each steak. Roll up and secure with toothpicks.

Grill the rolled steaks for about 35 minutes on the preheated grill, turning once in a while, until they reach your desired doneness. Take off the toothpicks before serving.

Nutrition ·

Calories: 163

Protein: 3 g

Sugar: 1 g

Fiber: 0.7 g

Carbohydrates: 45.6 g

Fat: 0.6g

Sodium: 87 mg

37. Eggplant Parmigiana Caponata

Preparation Time: 30 minutes

Cooking Time: 1hour 10 minutes

Servings: 8

Ingredients

1 cup olive oil, divided
1 eggplant, sliced into 1/2-inch rounds
2 red bell peppers, chopped
8 slices mozzarella cheese
1 small onion, chopped
2 cloves garlic, minced
1 (16 oz.) can stewed tomatoes, with juice
1 tbsp. chopped fresh basil
1 tbsp. chopped fresh oregano
1/4 cup balsamic vinegar
1/4 cup red wine vinegar
1/2 cup brown sugar
8 tbsps. Tomato paste
8 anchovy fillets, chopped (optional)
3 tbsps. Capers, chopped
1 tsp. salt
1 tsp. ground black pepper
1 cup grated Parmesan cheese

Directions

Set an oven to 175°C (350°F) and start preheating.
In a large heavy skillet, heat 1/2 cup of olive oil. Then sauté
the eggplant until each piece is saturated with oil. Line the

bottom of a 3-quart casserole dish with eggplant. Sauté red peppers until they are tender, then place into a layer on the eggplant in the casserole dish. Place mozzarella on top.

Heat the rest of the olive oil and cook garlic and onions until they are caramelized and browned lightly. Stir in oregano, basil, and stewed tomatoes and let it simmer for 5 minutes. Add tomato paste, brown sugar, red wine vinegar, and balsamic vinegar. Let it simmer for 10 minutes. Add capers and anchovy fillets, if using. Flavor with pepper and salt. Pour on the mozzarella cheese in the casserole dish. Scatter on the top of sauce with Parmesan cheese.

In the prepared oven, bake until the cheese melts, or for 20-25 minutes.

Nutrition

Calories: 288
Protein: 6 g
Sugar: 1.3 g
Fiber: 4 g

Carbohydrates: 43.6 g
Fat: 0.8g
Sodium: 98 mg

38. Smothered Sway

Preparation Time: 10 minutes

Cooking Time: 40 minutes

Servings: 5

Ingredients

5 (4 oz.) fillets sway fish   1 tsp. dried parsley
1/2 tsp. garlic powder   1/2 tsp. dried basil
2 tbsps. Lemon juice, or more to taste
Salt and ground black pepper to taste
1 cup shredded sharp Cheddar cheese
1 (15 oz.) can fire-roasted diced tomatoes

Directions

Preheat oven to 350°F (175°C).
In an 8x11-inch baking tray, place sway fish and pour lemon juice over it, seasoning with salt, pepper, garlic powder and parsley. Top with Cheddar cheese, fire-roasted tomatoes and basil.
Place tray in the preheated oven and bake for about 30 minutes until fish easily flakes using a fork.

Nutrition

Calories: 100   Carbohydrates: 21g
Protein: 1.8g   Fat: 2g
Sugar: 2.5g   Sodium: 56mg
Fiber: 0g

39. Chicken with Broccoli & Mushrooms

Preparation Time: 15 minutes

Cooking Time: 25 minutes

Servings: 6

Ingredients

3 tablespoons olive oil
6 garlic cloves, minced
¼ cup water
1-pound skinless, boneless chicken breast, cubed
Salt and ground black pepper, to taste

1 medium onion, chopped
2 cups fresh mushrooms, sliced
16 ounces small broccoli florets

Directions

Heat the oil in a large wok over medium heat and cook the chicken cubes for about 4–5 minutes.
With a slotted spoon, transfer the chicken cubes onto a plate.
In the same wok, add the onion and sauté for about 4–5 minutes.
Add the mushrooms and cook for about 4–5 minutes.
Stir in the cooked chicken, broccoli, and water, and cook (covered) for about 8–10 minutes, stirring occasionally.
Stir in salt and black pepper and remove from heat.
Serve hot.

Nutrition

Calories: 159
Protein: 2g
Sugar: 2.5g
Fiber: 0.3g

Carbohydrates: 40.3g
Fat: 2g
Sodium: 76mg

40. Shrimp with Kale

Preparation Time: 15 minutes

Cooking Time: 10 minutes

Servings: 4

Ingredients

3 tablespoons olive oil

1 medium onion, chopped

4 garlic cloves, chopped finely

1 fresh red chili, sliced

1-pound medium shrimp, peeled and deveined

1-pound fresh kale, tough ribs removed and chopped

¼ cup low-sodium chicken broth

Directions

In a large non-stick wok, heat 1 tablespoon of the oil over medium-high heat and cook the shrimp for about 2 minutes per side.

With a slotted spoon, transfer the shrimp onto a plate.

In the same wok, heat the remaining 2 tablespoons of oil over medium heat and sauté the garlic and red chili for about 1 minute.

Add the kale and broth and cook for about 4–5 minutes, stirring occasionally.

Stir in the cooked shrimp and cook for about 1 minute.

Serve hot.

Nutrition

Calories: 150

Carbohydrates: 34g

Protein: 1g

Fat: 0.3g

Sugar: 1g

Sodium: 93mg

Fiber: 0g

41. Rack of Lamb

Preparation Time: 15 minutes

Cooking Time: 30 minutes

Servings: 2

Ingredients

2 tbsps. All-purpose flour
1 cup white wine or chicken broth
1 tsp. grated lemon peel
1/2 tsp. dried rosemary, crushed
1 bay leaf
1 rack of lamb (1-1/2 lbs. and 8 ribs), trimmed

1 tsp. salt
1/2 tsp. pepper
2 tbsps. Butter
1 garlic clove, minced

Directions

In a shallow bowl, put pepper, salt and flour; coat lamb in flour mixture. Cook lamb in butter in a big skillet on medium high heat for 2 minutes per side; put onto a greased baking sheet. Bake without cover for 15-20 minutes at 375° till meat hits desired doneness (meat thermometer should read 170° for well-done, 160° for medium and 145° for medium-rare). Meanwhile, put bay leaf, rosemary, garlic, lemon peel and wine in skillet; boil. Cook for 8 minutes till liquid reduces by half. Take away lamb from oven; loosely cover with foil. Stand before slicing for 5 minutes; serve lamb with sauce.

Nutrition

Calories: 644
Protein: 1 g
Sugar: 0.2 g
Fiber: 0g

Carbohydrates: 34 g
Fat: 0.5g
Sodium: 64 mg

Chapter 10
Appetizer Recipes

42. Roasted Chickpeas

Preparation Time: 10 minutes

Cooking Time: 9 hours 20 minutes

Servings: 12

Ingredients

1 lb. dried chickpeas   2 tbsps. Olive oil
Kosher salt to taste

Directions

In a big container, put the chickpeas and pour a couple inches of cold water to cover, then allow it to stand for 8 hours to overnight.

Let the chickpeas drain and pat it dry.

Set an oven to preheat to 200°C (400°F).

In a bowl, toss together the salt, olive oil and chickpeas until coated evenly, then spread it on a baking tray in a single layer.

Let it roast in the preheated oven for about 40 minutes, mixing every 8 minutes, until the chickpeas become crisp and turns brown.

Toss the chickpeas with more salt and allow it to fully cool.

Nutrition ·

Calories: 507

Protein: 0.4g

Sugar: 0.5g

Fiber: 0.1g

Carbohydrates: 48g

Fat: 2g

Sodium: 27mg

43. Mango Salsa

Preparation Time: 15 minutes

Cooking Time: 1hour 15 minutes

Servings: 6

Ingredients

4 mangos - peeled, seeded, and diced
1 (15 oz.) can black beans, rinsed and drained
1 (10 oz.) can white shoepeg corn, drained
2 tbsps. Chopped fresh cilantro
1 lime, juiced
Salt and pepper to taste

Directions

Mix pepper, salt, lime juice, cilantro, corn, black beans and diced mango in a bowl.
Chill for at least 1 hour; serve.

Nutrition

Calories: 99
Protein: 1.7g
Sugar: 2g
Fiber: 0g

Carbohydrates: 32g
Fat: 2g
Sodium: 47mg

44. Grape Caterpillars

Preparation Time: 15 minutes

Cooking Time: 15 minutes

Servings: 4

Ingredients

20 green grapes
Skewers

1 tbsp. cream cheese, softened
10 miniature chocolate chips

Directions

Choose 5 nicest looking grapes.
Put on each one with 2 small dollops of cream cheese to make eyes and stick in mini chocolate chips for the pupils.
Thread 3-4 grapes lengthways onto a skewer, depending on the length of your skewers, followed by the grape with the eyes horizontally.
Repeat with other grapes.

Nutrition

Calories: 31
Protein: 4g
Sugar: 0.6g
Fiber: 1g

Carbohydrates: 32g
Fat: 2g
Sodium: 29mg

45. Crab Filled Deviled Eggs

Preparation Time: 20 minutes

Cooking Time: 20 minutes

Servings: 16

Ingredients

8 hard-boiled large eggs
2 tbsps. Lemon juice
1 tbsp. chopped green onion
1/4 tsp. hot pepper sauce
1 can (6 oz.) crabmeat, drained, flaked and cartilage removed

3 tbsps. Fat-free mayonnaise
4 tsps. Minced fresh tarragon
1/4 tsp. salt
1/8 tsp. cayenne pepper

Directions

Halve the eggs lengthwise.
Take out the yolks, then put aside the 4 yolks and egg whites
Mash the reserved yolks in a big bowl. Stir in cayenne, hot pepper sauce, salt, onion, tarragon, lemon juice and mayonnaise.
Mix in crab until well blended. Pipe or stuff it into egg whites, then chill it in the fridge until ready to serve.

Nutrition

Calories: 321
Protein: 2g
Sugar: 1g
Fiber: 0g

Carbohydrates: 23g
Fat: 1.7g
Sodium: 103mg

46. Cinnamon Toasties

Preparation Time: 10 minutes

Cooking Time: 20 minutes

Servings: 4

Ingredients

8 slices bread   1/4 cup reduced-fat cream cheese
3 tbsps. Sugar   Refrigerated butter-flavored spray
1-1/2 tsps. Ground cinnamon

Directions

Use a rolling pin to flatten bread.
Spread half of the slices with cream cheese on one side; put remaining bread on top.
Slice into four squares each. Spritz butter-flavored spray on both sides.
Mix cinnamon and sugar in a small bowl; include bread squares and flip to cover both sides.
Put on an ungreased baking sheet. Bake for 8-10 minutes at 350° or until golden and puffed. Serve right away.

Nutrition

Calories: 231   Carbohydrates: 42g
Protein: 0.6g   Fat: 1g
Sugar: 0.3g   Sodium: 98mg
Fiber: 1g

47. Fusion Peach Salsa

Preparation Time: 5 minutes

Cooking Time: 5 minutes

Servings: 4

Ingredients

2 tsps. Chopped fresh cilantro   2 tbsps. Lime juice
2 tsps. Garlic chile paste   1/8 tsp. white pepper
2 (15 oz.) cans peaches, drained and chopped
2 green onions with tops, thinly sliced
1/4 tsp. Asian five-spice powder

Directions

Mix together lime juice, cilantro, green onion and peaches in a medium bowl, then combine in white pepper, garlic Chile paste and five-spice powder.
Chill with a cover until serving.

Nutrition

Calories: 103   Carbohydrates: 39g
Protein: 1g   Fat: 1g
Sugar: 1g   Sodium: 87mg
Fiber: 0g

48. Basil and Pesto Hummus

Preparation Time: 10 minutes

Cooking Time: 10 minutes

Servings: 5

Ingredients

1/2 cup basil leaves
1 tbsp. olive oil
1/2 tsp. soy sauce
1 clove garlic
1/2 tsp. balsamic vinegar
Salt and ground black pepper
1 (16 oz.) garbanzo beans (chickpeas), drained and rinsed

Directions

In a food processor, mix garlic, basil, and garbanzo beans, then pulse a few times.
Scrape down the sides of the processor bowl using a spatula. Pulse again while drizzling in the olive oil.
Stir in soy sauce and vinegar, and process until incorporated. Sprinkle pepper and salt to season.

Nutrition

Calories: 131
Protein: 0g
Sugar: 0.4g
Fiber: 0g
Carbohydrates: 56g
Fat: 0g
Sodium: 22mg

49. Sweet Potato Chips

Preparation Time: 5 minutes

Cooking Time: 15 minutes

Servings: 2

Ingredients

1 sweet potato, thinly sliced   2 tsps. Olive oil
Coarse sea salt

Directions

Mix olive oil and sweet potato slices in a big bowl and coat by tossing.
Place the sweet potato slices in one layer on a big plate that's microwave safe. Season using salt.
Cook until slightly browned, crisp, and dry in a microwave for 5 minutes.
Cool the chips on a plate then transfer to a bowl. Repeat steps with leftover sweet potato slices.

Nutrition

Calories 140
Protein: 3g
Sugar: 2.3g
Fiber: 0g

Carbohydrates: 64g
Fat: 1.3g
Sodium: 17mg

50. Mango Mania Salsa

Preparation Time: 30 minutes

Cooking Time: 40 minutes

Servings: 24

Ingredients

1 red onion, peeled and halved
12 mangos - peeled, seeded, and diced
1/2 head garlic, pressed
3 habanero peppers, seeded and minced
1 bunch fresh cilantro, chopped
2 tbsps. Apple cider vinegar
Salt to taste

Directions

Preheat outdoor grill to high heat.
Oil the grate lightly. Put onion onto grill.
Cook until blackened slightly.
Dice onion. In a mixing bowl, mix apple cider, cilantro, habanero, garlic and mango. Season with salt to taste.

Nutrition

Calories: 72
Protein: 3g
Sugar: 1g
Fiber: 1.4g

Carbohydrates: 34g
Fat: 2g
Sodium: 20mg

51. Marinated Mushrooms

Preparation Time: 15 minutes

Cooking Time: 25 minutes

Servings: 8

Ingredients

1 cup red wine
1/3 cup olive oil
2 cloves garlic, minced
1/4 tsp. dried oregano
1/2 tsp. salt
1/4 tsp. ground black pepper
1 lb. small fresh mushrooms, washed and trimmed

1/2 cup red wine vinegar
2 tbsps. Brown sugar
1 tsp. crushed red pepper flakes
1/4 cup red bell pepper, diced
1/4 cup chopped green onions

Directions

Mix together the mushrooms, red pepper flakes, bell pepper, garlic, sugar, oil, vinegar and wine in a saucepan on medium heat, then boil.
Put cover and put aside to let it cool.
Mix in pepper, salt, oregano and green onions once cooled.
Serve it at room temperature or chilled.

Nutrition

Calories: 212
Protein: 4g
Sugar: 2g
Fiber: 3g

Carbohydrates: 18g
Fat: 3g
Sodium: 107mg

52. Layered Creamy Taco Dip

Preparation Time: 20 minutes

Cooking Time: 20 minutes

Servings: 4

Ingredients

1/2 cup reduced-fat sour cream
1/4 cup fat-free mayonnaise
1 medium green pepper, diced
1 medium tomato, diced
2 cups shredded part-skim mozzarella cheese
1 package (8 oz.) fat-free cream cheese

2 tsps. Taco seasoning
1 cup taco sauce
3 green onions, chopped
Tortilla chips

Directions

Beat taco seasoning, mayonnaise, sour cream and cream cheese in a bowl till smooth. Transfer into a 12-inch round serving plate and spread.

Top off with taco sauce and spread. Sprinkle with tomato, onions, green pepper and mozzarella cheese.

Store in the fridge, covered, till serving. Serve with tortilla chips.

Nutrition

Calories: 211
Protein: 3g
Sugar: 1g
Fiber: 0g

Carbohydrates: 56g
Fat: 2g
Sodium: 26mg

53. Garlic Spinach Balls

Preparation Time: 25 minutes

Cooking Time: 40 minutes

Servings: 8

Ingredients

2 cups crushed seasoned stuffing
1 cup finely chopped onion
1/2 cup grated Parmesan cheese
1-1/2 tsps. dried thyme
1/4 tsp. pepper
2 packages (10 oz. each) frozen chopped spinach, thawed and squeezed dry
3/4 cup butter, melted
4 large eggs, beaten
1 garlic clove, minced
1/4 tsp. salt

Directions

Mix together the initial 9 ingredients in a big bowl.
Mix in spinach until combined. Roll it into 1-inch balls, then put it in a greased 15x10x1-inch baking pan.
Let it bake for 15-20 minutes at 350 degrees or until it turns golden brown in color.

Nutrition

Calories: 234
Protein: 3g
Sugar: 1g
Fiber: 1g
Carbohydrates: 63g
Fat: 0g
Sodium: 112mg

54. Mango Salsa

Preparation Time: 20 minutes

Cooking Time: 1 hour 20 minutes

Servings: 40

Ingredients

2 cups diced Roma tomatoes
1/2 cup diced onion
1/2 cup chopped fresh cilantro
1 tbsp. cider vinegar
1/2 tsp. black pepper

1 1/2 cups diced mango
1 tsp. white sugar
2 tbsps. Fresh lime juice
1/2 tsp. salt
2 cloves garlic, minced

Directions

In a bowl, stir together garlic, pepper, salt, cider vinegar, lime juice, cilantro, sugar, onion, mango and tomatoes, then chill about 1 hour before serving.

Nutrition

Calories: 251
Protein: 6g
Sugar: 0.8g
Fiber: 1g

Carbohydrates: 13.4g
Fat: 9.3g
Sodium: 37mg

55. Stuffed Dates

Preparation Time: 15 minutes

Cooking Time: 15 minutes

Servings: 10

Ingredients

3 oz. reduced-fat cream cheese   30 pitted dates
1/4 cup confectioners' sugar   2 tsps. grated orange zest

Directions

Beat the orange zest, confectioner's sugar and cream cheese in a small bowl until combined.
Make a slit in the middle of each date carefully, then fill it with the cream cheese mixture. Put cover and let it chill in the fridge for a minimum of 1 hour prior to serving.

Nutrition

Calories: 200
Protein: 6g
Sugar: 1.6g
Fiber: 1g

Carbohydrates: 6.4g
Fat: 7.1g
Sodium: 183mg

56. Feta-spinach Melts

Preparation Time: 20 minutes

Cooking Time: 25 minutes

Servings: 10

Ingredients

1/2 cup crumbled feta cheese
1 plum tomatoes, seeded, chopped
1/4 cup finely chopped red onion
3 tbsps. fat-free mayonnaise
3 tbsps. fat-free sour cream
20 slices French baguette (1/2 inch thick)
3 packages (6 oz. each) fresh baby spinach, chopped

1 tsp. water
1/2 tsp. salt
1/2 tsp. dill weed
1 garlic clove, minced

Directions

Mix spinach with water in a big microwave-safe bowl. Cover and microwave at high heat until spinach is diminished, for 1 1/2 to 2 minutes, stir twice then drain and squeeze.
Mix in the dill weed, salt, garlic, sour cream, mayonnaise, onion, tomato, and feta cheese; put aside.
Lay bread on a baking tray. Put the tray 4 inches away from the heat source and broil until bread is toasted slightly, for 1 to 2 minutes. Add about 1 tbsp. of the spinach mixture over each bread. Broil for 3 to 4 more minutes until cooked through.

Nutrition

Calories: 156
Protein: 3.8g
Sugar: 8g
Fiber: 3g

Carbohydrates: 11.5g
Fat: 11.2g
Sodium: 360mg

Chapter 11
Dessert Recipes

57. Apricot Noodle Kugel

Preparation Time: 25 minutes

Cooking Time: 1 hour 10 minutes

Servings: 12

Ingredients

1 (8 oz.) package wide egg noodles
1/4 cup butter, softened
1 (3 oz.) package cream cheese
1/2 cup golden raisins (optional)
1 1/2 cups cornflake crumbs
1/2 cup butter, softened
1 tsp. vanilla extract

1/2 cup white sugar
1 tsp. vanilla extract
3 eggs, beaten
1 cup apricot nectar
1 cup milk
1/4 cup white sugar
1 tsp. ground cinnamon

Directions

Preheat oven to 175°C (350°F). Lightly spread cooking spray over a 9x9 inch baking pan.

Bring a big saucepan of slightly salted water to a boil. Mix in egg noodles and cook until al dente, about 8 to 10 minutes; let dry.

Blend vanilla, 1/2-cup sugar, eggs, cream cheese, 1/4-cup butter with egg noodles carefully in a medium bowl. Mix in milk and nectar apricot nectar. Blend in the raisins. Move to the prepared baking pan.

Blend cinnamon, remaining vanilla, 1/4 cup sugar, 1/2 cup butter and cornflake crumbs in a separate medium bowl. Pour evenly over the egg noodle blend.

Bake for 45 minutes.

Nutrition

Calories: 230
Protein: 2g
Sugar: 2g
Fiber: 0g

Carbohydrates: 11.6g
Fat: 7.2g
Sodium: 53mg

58. Honey Baked Apples

Preparation Time: 15 minutes

Cooking Time: 1 hour 15 minutes

Servings: 6

Ingredients

6 green apples
2 1/4 cups water
3 tbsps. Honey

1 1/2 cups fresh cranberries
3/4 cup packed brown sugar
6 scoops vanilla ice cream

Directions

Set an oven to preheat to 175°C (350°F).

Take off the peel from the top third of each apple, then core. In a baking dish, put the apples and put as many cranberries as you can fit to fill the core holes.

In a lesser saucepan, mix the honey, brown sugar and water, then boil and mix from time to time, until the honey and sugar dissolves, if needed. When it boils, pour the mixture on top of the apples.

Bake for an hour and moisten it using the juices every 15-20 minutes. Serve together with vanilla ice cream.

Nutrition

Calories: 252
Cholesterol: 9mg
Protein: 1.3g

Total Carbohydrate: 61g
Total Fat: 2.3g
Sodium: 27mg

59. Chewy Date Cookies

Preparation Time: 15 minutes

Cooking Time: 30 minutes

Servings: 2

Ingredients

1/3 cup butter, softened
1 egg
2/3 cup whole wheat flour
1-1/2 tsps. baking powder
1/2 tsp. ground nutmeg
1/4 cup fat-free milk

2/3 cup packed brown sugar
3/4 cup all-purpose flour
2 tsps. grated lemon peel
1/2 tsp. ground cinnamon
1/4 tsp. salt
1 cup chopped dates

Directions

Whip butter with brown sugar in a bowl. Put in egg; stir well.
Mix the salt, nutmeg, cinnamon, baking powder, lemon peel
and flours; alternately put into whipped mixture with milk,
mixing well after each addition. Mix in dates.
Put by heaping tablespoonfuls 2 inches apart onto baking
trays, ungreased. Bake for 13-15 minutes at 325° or until
golden brown. Take out to wire racks to cool. Put in an
airtight container to store.

Nutrition

Calories: 280
Protein: 4.7g
Sugar: 0.8g
Fiber: 1g

Carbohydrates: 13.9g
Fat: 3g
Sodium: 136mg

60. Blueberry Betty

Preparation Time: 10 minutes

Cooking Time: 30 minutes

Servings: 2

Ingredients

3/4 cup fat-free evaporated milk   2 eggs, lightly beaten
1/3 cup sugar   1 tsp. vanilla extract
1/2 tsp. ground cinnamon   1/4 tsp. salt
1 cup fresh or frozen blueberries   Dash ground nutmeg
2 slices raisin bread, toasted and cubed

Directions

Beat the salt, cinnamon, vanilla, sugar substitute, milk and eggs in a bowl, then mix in blueberries.
Pour it in 2 cooking spray coated 1-cup baking dishes. Put toasted cubes on top and sprinkle nutmeg on top. Let it bake for 20 to 25 minutes at 350 degrees or until it becomes bubbly.

Nutrition

Calories: 69   Carbohydrates: 15g
Protein: 1g   Fat: 0g
Sugar: 0.6g   Sodium: 36mg
Fiber: 1g

61. Baked Banana Boats

Preparation Time: 10 minutes

Cooking Time: 20 minutes

Servings: 4

Ingredients

4 medium bananas, unpeeled   1/4 cup chopped pecans
1/4 cup granola without raisins
1/2 cup unsweetened crushed pineapple, drained
4 tsps. miniature semisweet chocolate chips

Directions

Slice every banana into lengthwise, approximately half an inch deep and leave both ends with half an inch uncut. In a 12-inch square of foil, put each banana, then shape and crimp the foil surrounding the bananas so that they will sit flat.

Lightly pull every banana peel open to form a pocket. Fill chocolate chips, pecans, granola and pineapple on the pockets.

Put it on a baking tray and let it bake for 10 to 12 minutes at 350 degrees, until the chips become soft.

Nutrition

Calories: 220 calories   Total Carbohydrate: 40 g
Cholesterol: 0 mg   Total Fat: 8 g
Fiber: 5 g   Protein: 4 g
Sodium: 4 mg

62. Raspberry Cream Cake

Preparation Time: 20 minutes

Cooking Time: 50 minutes

Servings: 14

Ingredients

1 package yellow cake mix
2 tbsps. Unsweetened applesauce
1-1/3 cups cold fat-free milk
3/4 tsp. vanilla extract
1/4 tsp. baking soda
1-1/3 cups water
4 large egg whites
1 tbsp. light corn syrup
1 package (1 oz.) sugar-free instant vanilla pudding mix
1-1/2 cups fresh raspberries, divided
1/2 cup fat-free hot fudge ice cream topping

Directions

Mix baking soda and cake mix in a large bowl. Add applesauce, egg whites, and water; whisk for half a minute at low speed. Whisk for 2 minutes at medium speed.

Add into 2 greased 9-inch round baking pans. Bake at 350 degrees until a toothpick comes out clean when inserted into the center, for 28-32 minutes. Let it cool for 10 minutes, then transfer from the pans onto wire racks to cool completely.

For the filling: Beat vanilla, pudding mix, and milk for 2 minutes in a large bowl; allow to stand until soft set, for 2 minutes.

On a serving plate, arrange 1 cake layer. Spread the pudding mixture over; dust with 3/4 cup of the raspberries.

Add the rest of the cake layer on top. Mix corn syrup and

ice cream topping; whisk until smooth. Apply over the top of the cake and allow the glaze to drip over the sides. Top with the rest of berries.

Nutrition

Calories: 215 calories
Cholesterol: 0 mg
Fiber: 2 g
Sodium: 388 mg

Total Carbohydrate: 42 g
Total Fat: 4 g
Protein: 4 g

63. Pineapple Almond Bars

Preparation Time: 10 minutes

Cooking Time: 35 minutes

Servings: 2

Ingredients

3/4 cup all-purpose flour
1/3 cup packed brown sugar
1/2 tsp. almond extract
1 cup pineapple preserves

3/4 cup quick-cooking oats
5 tbsps. Reduced-fat butter
3 tbsps. Sliced almonds

Directions

Mix the brown sugar, oats and flour in a food processor. Put on cover and process until combined. Add extract and butter, put on cover and pulse until it becomes crumbly. Take out half a cup of crumb mixture into a bowl, then mix in sliced almonds.

Press the leftover crumb mixture in a cooking spray coated 9-inch square baking pan. Spread the conserves on top of the crust, then sprinkle the reserved crumb mixture on top. Let it bake for 25 to 30 minutes at 350 degrees or until it turns golden. Allow to cool on a wire rack.

Nutrition

Calories: 166 calories
Cholesterol: 0 mg
Fiber: 1 g
Sodium: 39 mg

Total Carbohydrate: 34 g
Total Fat: 4 g
Protein: 2 g

64. Berry Shortcakes

Preparation Time: 15 minutes

Cooking Time: 20 minutes

Servings: 4

Ingredients

2 cups sliced fresh strawberries, divided
1/2 tsp. grated lime zest
2 individual round sponge cakes
Whipped topping, optional

2 tbsps. sugar
1/2 tsp. cornstarch
2 tbsps. water
2 cups blueberries

Directions

Mix cornstarch and sugar in small saucepan; mix water in. Add 1 cup strawberries and mash mixture; boil.
Mix and cook till thick for 1-2 minutes; take off heat. Mix lime zest in. Put in small bowl; refrigerate till chilled, covered.
Crosswise, cut sponge cakes in half; trim each so it fits in bottoms of 4 1/2-pint wide mouth canning jars. Mix leftover strawberries and blueberries in small bowl; put on cakes. Put sauce on top. Serve with whipped topping if desired.

Nutrition

Calories: 124 calories
Cholesterol: 10 mg
Fiber: 3 g
Sodium: 67 mg

Total Carbohydrate: 29 g
Total Fat: 1 g
Protein: 2 g

65. Orange Cashew Bars

Preparation Time: 25 minutes

Cooking Time: 40 minutes

Servings: 2

Ingredients

4 oz. reduced-fat cream cheese
1/4 cup packed brown sugar
2 tsps. vanilla extract

1/2 cup confectioners' sugar
1 large egg yolk
1-1/2 cups all-purpose flour

Filling:
1 cup packed brown sugar
1 large egg
2 tsps. vanilla extract
1/4 tsp. salt
1-1/2 cups salted cashews, coarsely chopped

3 large egg whites
3 tbsps. all-purpose flour
1/2 tsp. orange extract

Icing:
3/4 cup confectioners' sugar
1 tsp. grated orange zest

4 tsps. orange juice

Directions

Preheat the oven to 350°. Whisk sugars and cream cheese in a big bowl till smooth. Whisk in vanilla and egg yolk. Slowly mix in flour.

Force dough 1/4 in. up sides and onto bottom of a sprayed with cooking spray 13x9-inch baking pan. Bake till edges are light brown, about 15 to 20 minutes. Allow to cool on a wire rack for 10 minutes.

For filling, whisk salt, extracts, flour, egg, egg whites, and brown sugar in a big bowl till smooth. Mix in cashews. Put into crust. Bake till set, about 15 to 20 minutes more.

Allow to cool fully in pan on a wire rack. Combine icing ingredients in a small bowl; sprinkle on top. Slice into bars.

Nutrition

Calories: 145 calories

Cholesterol: 17 mg

Fiber: 0 g

Sodium: 98 mg

Total Carbohydrate: 21 g

Total Fat: 5 g

Protein: 3 g

66. Mock Ice Cream Sandwiches

Preparation Time: 15 minutes

Cooking Time: 15 minutes

Servings: 8

Ingredients

2 cups fat-free whipped topping
1/2 cup miniature semisweet chocolate chips
8 whole chocolate graham crackers

Directions

Mix together the chocolate chips and whipped topping in a bowl. Cut or break the graham crackers in 1/2. Spread the beaten topping mixture on top of the 1/2 of crackers and put the leftover crackers on top.
Use plastic to wrap it and let it freeze for a minimum of 1 hour.

Nutrition

Calories: 180 calories
Cholesterol: 0 mg
Fiber: 1 g
Sodium: 88 mg

Total Carbohydrate: 28 g
Total Fat: 7 g
Protein: 2 g

Chapter 12
Dinner Recipes

67. Green Goddess

Preparation Time: 15 minutes

Cooking Time: 1 hour 15 minutes

Servings: 8

Ingredients

3/4 cup sour cream

2 cloves garlic, minced

2 tsps. chopped tarragon

2 anchovy fillets

Salt and ground black pepper to taste

3/4 cup mayonnaise

1/4 cup fresh parsley leaves

1 tbsp. lemon juice

1/4 cup minced fresh chives

Directions

In a food processor or blender, process garlic, lemon juice, sour cream, anchovy fillets, parsley, tarragon, and mayonnaise until creamy and smooth.

Place the blended mixture in a bowl and stir in the minced chives gently.

Season it with pepper and salt.

Store it inside the refrigerator for at least 60 minutes before serving.

Nutrition

· ·

Calories: 164

Protein: 1.4g

Sugar: 0.3g

Fiber: 1g

Carbohydrates: 33g

Fat: 2g

Sodium: 43mg

68. Sage Carrots

Preparation Time: 10 minutes

Cooking Time: 30 minutes

Servings: 4

Ingredients

2 tsps. sweet paprika
2 tbsps. olive oil
1/4 tsp. black pepper

1 tbsp. chopped sage
1 lb. peeled and cubed carrots
1 chopped red onion

Directions

In a baking pan, combine the carrots with the oil and the other ingredients, toss and bake at 380 0F for 30 minutes. Divide between plates and serve.

Nutrition

Calories: 200
Protein: 4g
Sugar: 3g
Fiber: 1g

Carbohydrates: 56g
Fat: 3g
Sodium: 36mg

69. Hearty Cashew and Almond Butter

Preparation Time: 5 minutes

Cooking Time: 12 minutes

Servings: 1

Ingredients

1 cup almonds, blanched
2 tablespoons coconut oil

1/3 cup cashew nuts
1/3 teaspoon cinnamon

Directions

Pre-heat your oven to 350 degrees F.
Bake almonds and cashews for 12 minutes.
Let them cool.
Transfer to food processor and add remaining ingredients.
Add oil and keep blending until smooth.
Serve and enjoy!

Nutrition

Calories: 205
Protein: 6g
Sugar: 1g
Fiber: 0g

Carbohydrates: 34g
Fat: 1g
Sodium: 102mg

70. Shrimp and Endives

Preparation Time: 5 minutes

Cooking Time: 12 minutes

Servings: 4

Ingredients

2 tablespoons avocado oil   2 spring onions, chopped
2 endives, shredded   1 tablespoon balsamic vinegar
1 tablespoon chives, minced
A pinch of sea salt and black pepper
1-pound shrimp, peeled and deveined

Directions

Heat up a pan with the oil over medium-high heat, add the spring onions, endives and chives, stir and cook for 4 minutes.
Add the shrimp and the rest of the ingredients, toss, cook over medium heat for 8 minutes more, divide into bowls and serve.

Nutrition

Calories: 191   Carbohydrates: 11.3g
Protein: 1g   Fat: 2g
Sugar: 3g   Sodium: 212mg
Fiber: 4g

71. Coriander Snapper Mix

Preparation Time: 5 minutes

Cooking Time: 20 minutes

Servings: 4

Ingredients

2 tablespoons olive oil
2 garlic cloves, minced
1 tomato, cubed
1 zucchini, cubed
4 snapper fillets, boneless, skinless and cubed

1 tablespoon coriander, chopped
½ teaspoon cumin, ground
A pinch of salt and black pepper
½ teaspoon rosemary, dried

Directions

Heat up a pan with the oil over medium-high heat, add the garlic, tomato and zucchini and cook for 5 minutes.
Add the fish and the other ingredients, toss, cook the mix for 15 minutes more, divide it into bowls and serve.

Nutrition

Calories: 251
Protein: 7g
Sugar: 1.3g
Fiber: 2g

Carbohydrates: 14g
Fat: 4g
Sodium: 24mg

72. Masala Scallops

Preparation Time: 10 minutes

Cooking Time: 20 minutes

Servings: 4

Ingredients

A pinch of salt and black pepper
¼ teaspoon cinnamon powder
1 teaspoon garam masala
1 teaspoon coriander, ground
2 tablespoons cilantro, chopped
2 tablespoons olive oil
2 jalapenos, chopped
1-pound sea scallops
1 teaspoon cumin, ground

Directions

Heat up a pan with the oil over medium heat, add the jalapenos, cinnamon and the other ingredients except the scallops and cook for 10 minutes.
Add the rest of the ingredients, toss, cook for 10 minutes more, divide into bowls and serve.

Nutrition

Calories: 281
Protein: 17g
Sugar: 3g
Fiber: 0g
Carbohydrates: 11g
Fat: 4g
Sodium: 103mg

73. Tuna and Tomatoes

Preparation Time: 5 minutes

Cooking Time: 20 minutes

Servings: 4

Ingredients

1 yellow onion, chopped   1 tablespoon olive oil
1 cup tomatoes, chopped   1 red pepper, chopped
1 teaspoon sweet paprika   1 tablespoon coriander, chopped
1-pound tuna fillets, boneless, skinless and cubed

Directions

Heat up a pan with the oil over medium heat, add the onions and the pepper and cook for 5 minutes.
Add the fish and the other ingredients, cook everything for 15 minutes, divide between plates and serve.

Nutrition

Calories: 154   Carbohydrates: 14g
Protein: 7g   Fat: 4g
Sugar: 1g   Sodium: 76mg
Fiber: 1g

74. Scallops with Almonds and Mushrooms

Preparation Time: 5 minutes

Cooking Time: 10 minutes

Servings: 4

Ingredients

1-pound scallops
4 scallions, chopped
½ cup mushrooms, sliced
1 cup coconut cream

2 tablespoons olive oil
A pinch of salt and black pepper
2 tablespoon almonds, chopped

Directions

Heat up a pan with the oil over medium heat, add the scallions and the mushrooms and sauté for 2 minutes.
Add the scallops and the other ingredients, toss, cook over medium heat for 8 minutes more, divide into bowls and serve.

Nutrition

Calories: 322
Protein: 21g
Sugar: 6g
Fiber: 2g

Carbohydrates: 8.1g
Fat: 23g;
Sodium: 361mg

75. Ginger Mushrooms

Preparation Time: 10 minutes

Cooking Time: 20 minutes

Servings: 4

Ingredients

1-pound mushrooms, sliced
1 tablespoon ginger, grated
2 tablespoons balsamic vinegar
A pinch of salt and black pepper
2 tablespoons walnuts, chopped

1 yellow onion, chopped
1 tablespoon olive oil
2 garlic cloves, minced
1/4 cup lime juice

Directions

Heat up a pan with the oil over medium-high heat, add the onion and the ginger and sauté for 5 minutes.
Add the mushrooms and the other ingredients, toss, cook over medium heat for 15 minutes more, divide between plates and serve.

Nutrition

Calories: 120
Protein: 5g
Sugar: 1g
Fiber: 1g

Carbohydrates: 4g
Fat: 2g
Sodium: 20mg

76. Rosemary Endives

Preparation Time: 10 minutes

Cooking Time: 0 minutes

Servings: 4

Ingredients

2 tbsps. olive oil

2 halved endives

½ tsp. turmeric powder

1 tsp. dried rosemary

¼ tsp. black pepper

Directions

In a baking pan, combine the endives with the oil and the other ingredients, toss gently, introduce in the oven and bake at 400 0F for 20 minutes.

Divide between plates and serve.

Nutrition

Calories: 66

Protein: 0.3g

Sugar: 1.3g

Fiber: 2g

Carbohydrates: 1.2g

Fat: 2g

Sodium: 113mg

77. Kale Sauté

Preparation Time: 10 minutes

Cooking Time: 10 minutes

Servings: 4

Ingredients

1 chopped red onion
2 tbsps. olive oil
1 tbsp. chopped cilantro
2 minced garlic cloves

3 tbsps. Coconut amines
1 lb. torn kale
1 tbsp. lime juice

Directions

Heat up a pan with the olive oil over medium heat, add the onion and the garlic and sauté for 5 minutes.
Add the kale and the other ingredients, toss, cook over medium heat for 10 minutes, divide between plates and serve.

Nutrition

Calories: 200
Protein: 6g
Sugar: 1.6g
Fiber: 1g

Carbohydrates: 6.4g
Fat: 7.1g
Sodium: 183mg

78. Roasted Beets

Preparation Time: 10 minutes

Cooking Time: 30 minutes

Servings: 4

Ingredients

2 minced garlic cloves
4 peeled and sliced beets
2 tbsps. olive oil

1/4 tsp. black pepper
1/4 c. chopped walnuts
1/4 c. chopped parsley

Directions

In a baking dish, combine the beets with the oil and the other ingredients, toss to coat, introduce in the oven at 420 0F, and bake for 30 minutes.
Divide between plates and serve.

Nutrition

Calories: 156
Protein: 3.8g
Sugar: 8g
Fiber: 3g

Carbohydrates: 11.5g
Fat: 11.2g
Sodium: 360mg

79. Minty Tomatoes and Corn

Preparation Time: 5 minutes

Cooking Time: 0 minutes

Servings: 4

Ingredients

2 c. corn
2 tbsps. chopped mint
1/4 tsp. black pepper

1 tbsp. rosemary vinegar
1 lb. sliced tomatoes
2 tbsps. olive oil

Directions

In a salad bowl, combine the tomatoes with the corn and the other ingredients, toss and serve.
Enjoy!

Nutrition

Calories: 230
Protein: 2g
Sodium: 53mg

Carbohydrates: 11.6g
Fat: 7.2g   Sugar: 2g
Fiber: 0g

80. Pesto Green Beans

Preparation Time: 10 minutes

Cooking Time: 0 minutes

Servings: 4

Ingredients

2 tbsps. olive oil
Juice of 1 lemon
¼ tsp. black pepper
1 lb. trimmed and halved green beans

2 tsps. sweet paprika
2 tbsps. basil pesto
1 sliced red onion

Directions

Heat up a pan with the oil over medium-high heat, add the onion, stir and sauté for 5 minutes.
Add the beans and the rest of the ingredients, toss, cook over medium heat for 10 minutes, divide between plates and serve.

Nutrition

Calories: 280
Protein: 4.7g
Sugar: 0.8g
Fiber: 1g

Carbohydrates: 13.9g
Fat: 3g;
Sodium: 136mg

Chapter 13
Dips and Spreads Recipes

81. Spicy Bean Salsa

Preparation Time: 10 minutes

Cooking Time: 8 hours 10 minutes

Servings: 12

Ingredients

1 (15oz.) can black-eyed peas   1/2 cup chopped onion
1 cup Italian-style salad dressing   1/2 tsp. garlic salt
1 (15oz.) can whole kernel corn   1 (15oz.) can black beans
1/2 cup chopped green bell pepper
1 (4oz.) can diced jalapeno peppers
1 (14.5oz.) can diced tomatoes, drained

Directions

Mix tomatoes, jalapeno peppers, green bell pepper, onion, corn, black beans and black-eyed beans in a medium bowl. Season using garlic salt and Italian-style salad dressing; stir well.

Nutrition

Calories: 155   Total Carbohydrate: 20.4 g
Cholesterol: 0 mg   Total Fat: 6.4 g
Protein: 5 g   Sodium: 949 mg

82. Spicy Chili-cheese Dip

Preparation Time: 15 minutes

Cooking Time: 30 minutes

Servings: 12

Ingredients

2 (16 oz.) cans refried beans 1 (15 oz.) can chili
1 (8 oz.) package cream cheese, softened
1 (4 oz.) can chopped green chile peppers
1 cup shredded Cheddar cheese

Directions

Preheat an oven to 175°C/350°F.
Mix green Chile peppers, cream cheese, chili and refried beans well in stand mixer's bowl; put bean mixture in 9-in. square baking dish. Put Cheddar cheese on top.
In preheated oven, bake for 15 minutes till cheese melts and dip is bubbling.

Nutrition

Calories: 214
Cholesterol: 42 mg
Protein: 9.9 g

Total Carbohydrate: 16.9 g
Total Fat: 12.5 g
Sodium: 629 mg

83. Taco Bean Dip

Preparation Time: 10 minutes

Cooking Time: 1 hour 5 minutes

Servings: 12

Ingredients

1 (1 oz.) package taco seasoning mix   1/4 cup salsa
1/2 cup shredded Cheddar cheese   8 oz. sour cream
2 (11.5 oz.) cans condensed bean with bacon soup

Directions

Mix salsa, sour cream, seasoning mix and soup in a slow cooker. Put cheese on top; heat on low for 1 hour till cheese melts.

Nutrition

Calories: 132
Cholesterol: 15 mg
Protein: 5.3 g

Total Carbohydrate: 12.5 g
Total Fat: 6.7 g
Sodium: 639 mg

84. Vegetable Fajitas

Preparation Time: 20 minutes

Cooking Time: 30 minutes

Servings: 4

Ingredients

8 (8 inch) flour tortillas
1 red onion, thinly sliced
1 tsp. ground cumin
1/4 cup chopped fresh cilantro
1 cup shredded Monterey Jack cheese
1 green bell pepper, seeded and sliced into strips
1 red bell pepper, seeded and sliced into strips
1 yellow squash, halved and sliced into strips

2 tbsps. vegetable oil
1 tsp. minced garlic
1/2 tsp. salt
1/2 cup salsa

Directions

Use aluminum foil to wrap tortillas; put in oven. Put heat to 175°C/350°F. Bake till thoroughly heated for 15 minutes.
Heat oil in 10-in. skillet on medium high heat. Add green and red peppers, garlic and onions; mix to coat in oil. Cover; lower heat to medium. Cook for 5 minutes. Mix squash into veggies. Mix salt, cumin and salsa in; cover. Cook for 5 minutes.
Evenly put veggie mixture down centers of warm tortillas. Sprinkle cilantro and cheese; roll tortillas up.

Nutrition

Calories: 531
Cholesterol: 25 mg
Protein: 17.6 g

Total Carbohydrate: 64.7 g
Total Fat: 22.8 g
Sodium: 1111 mg

85. Spice Cookies with Pumpkin Dip

Preparation Time: 20 minutes

Cooking Time: 30 minutes

Servings: 8

Ingredients

1-1/2 cups butter, softened
2 large eggs
4 cups all-purpose flour
2 tsps. ground cinnamon
1 tsp. ground cloves
Additional granulated sugar

2 cups granulated sugar
1/2 cup molasses
4 tsps. baking soda
1 tsp. ground ginger
1 tsp. salt

Pumpkin Dip:
2 cups canned pumpkin pie mix
1/2 to 1 tsp. ground cinnamon
1 package (8 oz.) cream cheese, softened

2 cups confectioners' sugar
1/2 tsp. ground ginger

Directions

Cream granulated sugar and butter until fluffy and light. Whisk in molasses and eggs. Mix together the following 6 ingredients, add to the creamed mixture and stir thoroughly. Refrigerate overnight.

Form into balls, about 1/2-inch each, roll in extra sugar. Put on non-oiled cookie sheets, about 2-inch separately. Bake at 375° for 6 minutes until starting to turn brown. Let cool for 2 minutes, and then transfer onto a wire rack.

To prepare the dip, whisk cream cheese until smooth. Whisk in pumpkin pie mix. Add ginger, cinnamon, and confectioners' sugar; stir thoroughly. Enjoy with cookies. Chill leftover dip.

Nutrition ·

Calories: 108

Cholesterol: 18 mg

Fiber: 0 g

Sodium: 147 mg

Total Carbohydrate: 16 g

Total Fat: 5 g

Protein: 1 g

86. Shrimp Dip With Cream Cheese

Preparation Time: 10 minutes

Cooking Time: 10 minutes

Servings: 8

Ingredients

1 package (8 oz.) cream cheese
1 tsp. Worcestershire sauce
Dash white pepper
1 tbsp. finely chopped onion
1 can (6 oz.) small shrimp, rinsed and drained

1-1/2 tsps. lemon juice
1/8 tsp. salt
Assorted crackers

Directions

Combine pepper, salt, Worcestershire sauce, lemon juice and cream cheese in a small bowl then mix well until texture becomes smooth.
Add in the onion and shrimp. Place inside the refrigerator before serving time. Pair with crackers.

Nutrition

Calories: 59
Cholesterol: 43 mg
Fiber: 0 g
Sodium: 277 mg

Total Carbohydrate: 1 g
Total Fat: 4 g
Protein: 5 g

87. Amaretto-peach Cheese Spread

Preparation Time: 10 minutes

Cooking Time: 10 minutes

Servings: 16

Ingredients

1 jar (18 oz.) peach preserves   2 tbsps. Amaretto
1 cup finely chopped pecans   Gingersnap cookies
2 packages (8 oz. each) cream cheese, softened

Directions

On a serving plate, put cream cheese. Mix preserves, Amaretto, and pecans together, scoop over cream cheese. Enjoy with gingersnap cookies.

Nutrition

Calories: 233   Total Carbohydrate: 23 g
Cholesterol: 31 mg   Total Fat: 15 g
Fiber: 1 g   Protein: 3 g
Sodium: 84 mg

88. Blue Cheese Spread

Preparation Time: 15 minutes

Cooking Time: 15 minutes

Servings: 2

Ingredients

3 shallots, finely chopped
1/2 cup sour cream
1/4 tsp. salt
1/2 cup chopped walnuts, toasted
2 cups (8 oz.) crumbled blue cheese
2 packages (8 oz. each) cream cheese, softened

2 tsps. butter
2 tbsps. Cognac or brandy
1/4 tsp. white pepper
Assorted crackers

Directions

Sauté shallots with butter in a small skillet until softened. Take away from heat and allow to cool.

At the same time, mix together pepper, salt, Cognac, sour cream and cheeses in a big bow. Put in shallots and combine well. Use plastic wrap to line a 3-cup bowl, then spread cheese mixture in the prepared bowl. Cover and chill for a minimum of an hour.

Unmold onto a serving plate and decorate with walnuts. Serve along with crackers.

Nutrition

Calories: 141
Cholesterol: 33 mg
Fiber: 0 g
Sodium: 242 mg

Total Carbohydrate: 2 g
Total Fat: 12 g
Protein: 5 g

89. Quick Salsa

Preparation Time: 15 minutes

Cooking Time: 15 minutes

Servings: 8

Ingredients

4 large tomatoes, chopped
2 tbsps. minced fresh cilantro
1 garlic clove, minced
1/2 tsp. pepper
1/2 to 1 jalapeno pepper, seeded and minced
6 Anaheim peppers, roasted and peeled

3 green onions, sliced
1/3 cup olive oil
1/3 cup red wine vinegar
1 tsp. salt, optional

Directions

Mix together garlic, jalapeno, cilantro, onions, tomatoes and chilies in a big bowl.

Mix pepper, oil, vinegar and salt, if wanted, in a separate bowl then stir into the vegetable mixture. Cover and refrigerate for a minimum of 2 hours.

Nutrition

Calories: 27
Cholesterol: 0 mg
Fiber: 0 g
Sodium: 3 mg

Total Carbohydrate: 2 g
Total Fat: 2 g
Protein: 1 g

90. Vegetarian Pate

Preparation Time: 15 minutes

Cooking Time: 1 hour

Servings: 12

Ingredients

1 egg
1 large onion, chopped
20 thin wheat crackers
1 (15 oz.) can peas, drained
Salt and pepper to taste

3 tbsps. vegetable oil
2 cloves garlic, chopped
1/2 cup walnuts
1/2 tsp. seasoning salt

Directions

Get a small saucepan and put egg in it, then put cold water to cover. Make it boil, and once starts to boil, get the saucepan away from heat. Cover with a lid and maintain the egg in hot water for 10 to 12 minutes. Then get the egg from hot water, let it cool, then remove the shell and slice.

Place a skillet on the stove and turn on to low heat then put the oil to heat, stir in chopped onion. Continue stirring and cook until softened and turns to brown color. Stir in sliced garlic, and fry for 1 to 2 minutes. Get the mixture from the pan, then put aside to cool.

Use a food processor or a blender to finely chop the walnuts and wheat crackers. Add in the fried onion mixture, seasoning salt and peas. Stir in the egg, then mix until it becomes paste, you can add oil or water if needed to reach the consistency you want. Add pepper and salt to taste.

Nutrition ·

Calories: 103

Cholesterol: 16 mg

Protein: 2.8 g

Total Carbohydrate: 7.3 g

Total Fat: 7.4 g

Sodium: 137 mg

91. Mozzarella Dip

Preparation Time: 10 minutes

Cooking Time: 1 hour 10 minutes

Servings: 32

Ingredients

2 cups mayonnaise
1 cup shredded mozzarella cheese
2 tbsps. grated Parmesan cheese
1 dash garlic salt

1 cup sour cream
1 tsp. white sugar
1 tbsp. minced onion
1 dash seasoning salt

Directions

Combine mozzarella cheese, mayonnaise, garlic salt, seasoning salt, onion, sugar, sour cream and Parmesan cheese in a medium bowl and mix well then cover with a plastic wrap or a lid and place in the refrigerator for 1 hour then serve.

Nutrition

Calories: 125
Cholesterol: 11 mg
Protein: 1.3 g

Total Carbohydrate: 1 g
Total Fat: 13.1 g
Sodium: 126 mg

Chapter 14
Snack Recipes

92. Herbed Mixed Nuts

Preparation Time: 10 minutes

Cooking Time: 25 minutes

Servings: 12

Ingredients

1 tbsp. Worcestershire sauce   1 tbsp. butter, melted
2 tbsps. grated Parmesan cheese   ½ tsp. garlic salt
2 tsps. dried basil and/or oregano, crushed
3 cups walnuts, soy nuts, and/or almonds

Directions

Set an oven to preheat to 325° F. Mix together the garlic salt, herb, sauce and melted butter in a bowl. Add nuts and mix until coated. Use foil to line a 15x10x1-inch baking pan, then spread the nuts in the pan. Put parmesan on top, then stir until coated. Let it bake for 15 minutes, mixing two times. Allow it to cool.

Nutrition

Calories: 221
Protein: 2g
Sugar: 0.4g
Fiber: 0.7g

Carbohydrates: 16g
Fat: 2g
Sodium: 120mg

93. Cinnamon Graham Popcorn

Preparation Time: 10 minutes

Cooking Time: 30 minutes

Servings: 3

Ingredients

2-1/2 quarts popped popcorn
1-1/2 cups golden raisins
1 cup miniature marshmallows
1/4 cup packed brown sugar
1/2 tsp. ground ginger

2 cups Golden Grahams
1 cup chopped dates
1/3 cup butter, melted
2 tsps. ground cinnamon
1/2 tsp. ground nutmeg

Directions

Mix marshmallows, dates, raisins, cereal, and popcorn together in a big bowl.
Mix the rest of the ingredients together. Put on the popcorn mixture and mix to blend.
Put in two oiled 15x0x1-in. baking pans.
Bake without a cover at 250°, tossing 1 time, about 20 minutes. Preserve in an airtight container.

Nutrition

Calories: 243
Protein: 1g
Sugar: 2g
Fiber: 1g

Carbohydrates: 20g
Fat: 3g
Sodium: 34mg

94. Cheesy Ranch Chex

Preparation Time: 15 minutes

Cooking Time: 15 minutes

Servings: 26

Ingredients

9 cups Corn Chex®, Rice Chex® or Wheat Chex® cereal
2 cups bite-size pretzel twists
2 cups bite-size cheese crackers
3 tbsps. butter or margarine, melted
1 (1 oz.) package ranch dressing and seasoning mix
1/2 cup grated Parmesan cheese

Directions

Microwave butter in a big microwave-safe bowl without a cover on high setting until butter is melted, about a half minute.
Stir in crackers, pretzels and cereal until well-coated. Stir in cheese and dressing mix until coated evenly.
Microwave on high setting without cover for 3 minutes while stirring every minute. Scatter cereal mixture on foil or waxed paper to let it cool, for 15 minutes.
Keep in an airtight container.

Nutrition

Calories: 119
Protein: 3g
Sugar: 1g
Fiber: 4g

Carbohydrates: 23g
Fat: 2g
Sodium: 16mg

95. Almonds with Rosemary and Cayenne

Preparation Time: 10 minutes

Cooking Time: 15 minutes

Servings: 16

Ingredients

8 oz. unblanched almonds or pecan halves (about 2 cups)
1½ tsps. margarine or butter
1 tbsp. finely snipped fresh rosemary
1½ tsps. brown sugar
¼ to ½ tsp. salt
¼ tsp. ground red pepper

Directions

Set an oven to preheat to 350 degrees F. Spread the almonds or pecans on the baking tray in a single layer.
Let it bake for around 10 minutes or until it becomes aromatic and a bit toasted.
In the meantime, melt the margarine or butter in a medium saucepan on medium heat until it sizzles. Take it out of the heat. Stir in red pepper, salt, sugar and rosemary.
Add the nuts to the butter mixture and toss until coated.
Allow it to cool a bit prior to serving.

Nutrition

Calories: 80
Protein: 2g
Sugar: 2.1g
Fiber: 1g

Carbohydrates: 13g
Fat: 2g
Sodium: 59mg

96. Plum & Pistachio Snack

Preparation Time: 5 minutes

Cooking Time: 5 minutes

Servings: 1

Ingredients

¼ cup unsalted dry-roasted pistachios (measured in shell)
1 plum

Directions

Hull and serve pistachios together with plum.

Nutrition

Calories: 275
Protein: 3.5g
Sugar: 1g
Fiber: 3g

Carbohydrates: 23g
Fat: 1g
Sodium: 308mg

97. Peanut Butter & Pretzel Truffles

Preparation Time: 20 minutes

Cooking Time: 2 hours

Servings: 20

Ingredients

½ cup crunchy natural peanut butter
¼ cup finely chopped salted pretzels
½ cup milk chocolate chips, melted

Directions

In a small bowl, mix pretzels and peanut butter. Cool in the freezer for about 15 minutes until firm.
Roll peanut butter mixture into 20 balls (of about 1 tsp. each).
Transfer to a baking sheet that is lined with wax paper or parchment and the freeze for about 1 hour until very firm.
Roll the frozen balls in the melted chocolate.
Place in a fridge for about 30 minutes until chocolate is set.

Nutrition

Calories: 110
Protein: 12g
Sugar: 1.9g
Fiber: 3g

Carbohydrates: 43g
Fat: 1g
Sodium: 21mg

98. Mini Bagel Pizzas

Preparation Time: 10 minutes

Cooking Time: 20 minutes

Servings: 4

Ingredients

8 mini bagels, split   1/4 cup pizza sauce
1/3 cup shredded pizza cheese blend
16 slices turkey pepperoni

Directions

Set the oven to 220°C or 425°F. Use aluminum foil to line a baking sheet.
On prepared baking sheet, add bagels, with cut sides up. Scoop over each bagel half with a thin payer of pizza sauce, then sprinkle with pizza cheese. Put on each bagel with 2 pepperoni slices.
In the preheated oven, bake for 6 minutes, until pepperoni is browned a little bit and cheese is melted.

Nutrition

Calories: 381   Total Carbohydrate: 30.3 g
Cholesterol: 33 mg   Total Fat: 5.8 g
Protein: 13.9 g   Sodium: 788 mg

99. Candy Wraps

Preparation Time: 5 minutes

Cooking Time: 3 hours 5 minutes

Servings: 4

Ingredients

1 tsp. orange marmalade   1 tsp. pure maple syrup
1 (10 inch) whole wheat tortilla

Directions

On a clean surface or dinner plate, lay out the tortilla. Spread orange marmalade on one half while the other with maple syrup. Roll up the tortilla tightly, beginning at the end with the syrup and finishing with marmalade.
Hold it together with toothpicks, if necessary, or use plastic wrap to wrap. Chill for a couple of hours then cut into 1" pieces to serve.

Nutrition

Calories: 90
Cholesterol: 0 mg
Protein: 3 g

Total Carbohydrate: 24.4 g
Total Fat: 0.5 g
Sodium: 173 mg

100. Spicy Almonds

Preparation Time: 10 minutes

Cooking Time: 25 minutes

Servings: 4

Ingredients

1 tbsp. sugar
1 tsp. paprika
1/2 tsp. ground cumin
1/4 tsp. cayenne pepper
2-1/2 cups unblanched almonds

1-1/2 tsps. kosher salt
1/2 tsp. ground cinnamon
1/2 tsp. ground coriander
1 tbsp. canola oil

Directions

Mix the initial 7 ingredients in a small bowl. Mix oil and almonds in a separate small bowl.
Drizzle with spice mixture; coat by tossing.
In a 15x10x1-inch foil-lined baking pan sprayed with cooking spray, put the mixture. Bake till lightly browned for 15 to 20 minutes at 325°, mixing two times. Cool completely. Keep in an airtight container.

Nutrition

Calories: 230
Cholesterol: 0 mg
Fiber: 4 g
Sodium: 293 mg

Total Carbohydrate: 9 g
Total Fat: 20 g
Protein: 8 g

101. Rosemary Walnuts

Preparation Time: 10 minutes

Cooking Time: 20 minutes

Servings: 8

Ingredients

2 cups walnuts
1 tbsp. honey
1 tsp. salt

2 cloves garlic, minced
1 tbsp. extra-virgin olive oil
1 tbsp. minced fresh rosemary

Directions

Preheat your oven to 350°F (175°C). Prepare your baking pan and line it with a parchment paper.

In a clean bowl, combine honey, rosemary, salt, garlic, walnuts and olive oil. Mix until the walnuts are completely coated and transfer it into the prepared baking pan.

Bake the walnuts in the preheated oven for about 10 minutes or until lightly brown in color.

Nutrition

Calories: 188
Cholesterol: 0 mg
Protein: 3.9 g

Total Carbohydrate: 5.9 g
Total Fat: 18 g
Sodium: 291 mg

102. Gluten-free Snack Mix

Preparation Time: 10 minutes

Cooking Time: 25 minutes

Servings: 8

Ingredients

8 cups popped popcorn
1 package (5 oz.) dried cherries
1/3 cup honey

2 cups Koala Crisp cereal
1/3 cup butter, cubed
1/2 tsp. ground cinnamon

Directions

Mix together cherries, cereal and popcorn in a big ungreased roasting pan. Melt butter in a small saucepan. Put in cinnamon and honey, then cook and stir until heated through. Drizzle over popcorn mixture and toss to coat well.

Bake at 325 degrees for about 15 minutes while stirring after every 5 minutes. Allow to cool thoroughly. Store in airtight containers.

Nutrition

Calories: 110
Cholesterol: 8 mg
Fiber: 1 g
Sodium: 89 mg

Total Carbohydrate: 16 g
Total Fat: 5 g
Protein: 1 g

103. Cranberry Pretzels

Preparation Time: 15 minutes

Cooking Time: 15 minutes

Servings: 15

Ingredients

3/4 cup dried cranberries
1 cup warm milk
1-1/2 tsps. salt
2 quarts water
1 package (1/4 oz.) active dry yeast

2 tbsps. sugar, divided
3 tbsps. canola oil
3-1/2 to 4 cups all-purpose flour
1/3 cup unsweetened applesauce

Topping:
1/2 tsp. ground cinnamon
1 tbsp. sugar

1 egg white, beaten
Honey or cream cheese, optional

Directions

In a blender or food processor, put 1 tbsp. sugar, applesauce and dried cranberries. Put cover on and blend until chopped finely; set aside. Dissolve yeast with warm milk in a bowl. Put in the remaining sugar and allow to stand about 5 minutes. Put in salt, oil, sufficient flour and cranberry mixture to make a soft dough. Transfer to a surface coated lightly with flour, then knead dough for 6 to 8 minutes, until elastic and smooth. Put in a bowl coated with cooking spray and turn one time to coat the top. Cover and allow to rise on a warm area for 1 1/2 hours, until doubled in size.

Punch dough down then transfer onto a floured surface. Split dough into 15 balls, rolling each ball into a 14-in. rope and form into a pretzel shape.

Bring water in a big saucepan to a boil, then drop in pretzels, one at a time. Boil about 10 seconds on each side; take out of the water, using a slotted spoon. Transfer to paper towels to drain.

On baking sheets coated with cooking spray, place pretzels. Put cover on and allow to rise in warm area for 25 minutes, until puffy. Coat the surface with egg white. Mix sugar and cinnamon in, then sprinkle over tops of pretzels. Bake at 375° until turning golden brown, about 12 to 14 minutes. Serve with cream cheese or honey, if wanted.

Nutrition

Calories: 170
Cholesterol: 1 mg
Fiber: 1 g
Sodium: 248 mg

Total Carbohydrate: 31 g
Total Fat: 3 g
Protein: 4 g

104. Pumpkin Custard

Preparation Time: 30 minutes

Cooking Time: 35 minutes

Servings: 8

Ingredients

Custard
1½ teaspoons pumpkin pie spice   8 egg yolks
1 teaspoon vanilla   ½ cup sugar
1¾ cups (1 15-ounce can) pure pumpkin puree
1¾ cups heavy whipping cream

Topping
1 cup crushed gingersnap cookies
1 tablespoon melted butter

Whipped Cream
1 cup heavy whipping cream   1 tablespoon superfine sugar
½ teaspoon pumpkin pie spice

Garnish
8 whole gingersnap cookies

Directions

Preheat the oven to 350°F.
Separate the yolks from 8 eggs and whisk them together in a large mixing bowl until they are well blended and creamy.
Add the pumpkin, sugar, vanilla, heavy cream and pumpkin pie spice and whisk to combine.
Cook the custard mixture in a double boiler, stirring until it has thickened enough that it coats a spoon.

Pour the mixture into individual custard cups or an 8×8-inch baking pan and bake for about 20 minutes if using individual cups or 30–35 minutes for the baking pan, until it is set, and a knife inserted comes out clean.

While the custard is baking, make the topping by combining the crushed gingersnaps and melted butter. After the custard has been in the oven for 15 minutes, sprinkle the gingersnap mixture over the top.

When the custard has passed the clean knife test, remove from the oven and let cool to room temperature.

Whisk the heavy cream and pumpkin pie spice together with the caster sugar and beat just until it thickens.

Serve the custard with the whipped cream and garnish each serving with a gingersnap.

Nutrition

Calories: 255
Carbs: 25 g
Sodium: 877 mg

Fat: 35 g
Protein: 76 g

105. Baked Apple Dumplings

Preparation Time: 20 minutes

Cooking Time: 40 minutes

Servings: 2 to 4

Ingredients ·

1 cup sugar

1 egg, beaten

1 pinch ground nutmeg

4 Granny Smith apples, peeled, cored and halved

1 (17½ ounce) package frozen puff pastry, thawed

6 tablespoons dry breadcrumbs

2 teaspoons ground cinnamon

Vanilla ice cream for serving

Icing

1 cup confectioners' sugar

3 tablespoons milk

1 teaspoon vanilla extract

Pecan Streusel

2/3 Cup chopped toasted pecans

2/3 Cup all-purpose flour

2/3 Cup packed brown sugar

5 tablespoons melted butter

Directions ·

Preheat the oven to 425°F.

When the puff pastry has completely thawed, roll out each sheet to measure 12 inches by 12 inches. Cut the sheets into quarters.

Combine the sugar, breadcrumbs, cinnamon and nutmeg together in a small bowl.

Brush one of the pastry squares with some of the beaten egg. Add about 1 tablespoon of the breadcrumb mixture on top, then add half an apple, core side down, over the crumbs. Add another tablespoon of the breadcrumb mixture.

Seal the dumpling by pulling up the corners and pinching the pastry together until the seams are totally sealed. Repeat this process with the remaining squares.

Assemble the ingredients for the pecan streusel in a small bowl.

Grease a baking sheet, or line it with parchment paper. Place the dumplings on the sheet and brush them with a bit more of the beaten egg. Top with the pecan streusel.

Bake for 15 minutes, then reduce heat to 350°F and bake for 25 minutes more or until lightly browned.

Make the icing by combining the confectioners' sugar, vanilla and milk until you reach the proper consistency.

When the dumplings are done, let them cool to room temperature and drizzle them with icing before serving.

Nutrition

Calories: 145

Fat: 57 g

Carbs: 87 g

Protein: 66.9 g

Sodium: 529 mg

106. Peach Cobbler

Preparation Time: 10 minutes

Cooking Time: 45 minutes

Servings: 4

Ingredients

1¼ cups Bisques
½ cup melted butter
½ teaspoon cinnamon

1 cup milk
¼ teaspoon nutmeg
Vanilla ice cream, for serving

Filling
1 can peaches in syrup, drained

¼ cup sugar

Topping
½ cup brown sugar
½ teaspoon cinnamon

¼ cup almond slices
1 tablespoon melted butter

Directions

Preheat the oven to 375°F.

Grease the bottom and sides of an 8×8-inch pan.

Whisk together the Bisques, milk, butter, nutmeg and cinnamon in a large mixing bowl. When thoroughly combined, pour into the greased baking pan.

Mix together the peaches and sugar in another mixing bowl. Put the filling on top of the batter in the pan. Bake for about 45 minutes.

In another bowl, mix together the brown sugar, almonds, cinnamon, and melted butter. After the cobbler has cooked for 45 minutes, cover evenly with the topping and bake for an additional 10 minutes. Serve with a scoop of vanilla ice cream.

Nutrition . . . .

Calories: 168

Carbs: 15 g

Sodium: 436 mg

Fat: 76 g

Protein: 78.9 g

Chapter 15
Coffee Recipes

107. Irish coffee

Preparation Time: 15 minutes

Cooking Time: 0 minutes

Servings: 1

Ingredients

1.5 cl of cane sugar syrup   2 cl of fresh cream
3 cl of whiskey (bourbon, whiskey)   4 cl of coffee

Directions

Make the "Irish Coffee" recipe directly in the glass.
Heat the whiskey with the sugar (at low heat so as not to boil the whiskey) in a saucepan stirring. Prepare a black coffee and pour it over the hot and sweet whiskey, stir slightly. Pour everything into the formerly rinsed glass with warm water and coat the surface with lightly beaten cream, its ready! Savor without delay. To make your cream work better, place it in the freezer for 20 minutes before vigorously whipping it.
Despite some rumors of modern times, Irish coffee is not supposed to have the three separate floors. Other variants can be made with whipped cream instead of fresh cream, liquid cane sugar instead of powdered sugar or replace the traditional whiskey with whiskey or bourbon. Still, the original recipe is the one explained above.

Serve in a glass type "mug."
Add any grated chocolate to the cream.

Nutrition

Calories: 90

Fat: 2 g

Carbohydrates: 4 g

Protein: 14 g

108. Caramel coffee

Preparation Time: 15 minutes

Cooking Time: 0 minutes

Servings: 1

Ingredients

15 cl of milk
1 dash of cinnamon syrup

3 cl of caramel syrup
1 coffee

Directions

Make the recipe "Coffee Caramel."
Make a coffee (espresso). Heat the glass under hot water and pour the caramel syrup into the bottom of the glass. Heat the milk in another container until creamy foam and pour the warm milk gently on the syrup. Pour a few drops of cinnamon syrup and pour the coffee gently over the milk (use a spoon) until you get an extra layer...
Serve in a tumbler type glass.
Sprinkle with cinnamon powder.

Nutrition

Calories: 20
Carbohydrates: 4 g

Fat: 0 g
Protein: 1 g

109. Latte macchiato

Preparation Time: 15 minutes

Cooking Time: 0 minutes

Servings: 1

Ingredients

Coffee   20 cl of milk

Directions

Make the recipe "Latte macchiato" directly in the glass.
Beat the milk (preferably whole) with a whisk in a saucepan over the heat to obtain foam on the surface (or using the steam nozzle of your espresso machine).
Pour warm milk into a heat-resistant glass (thick walls), blocking the foam with a spatula.
Add the milk foam on the hot milk.
Finally, gently pour a strong espresso (sweetened according to taste) on the frothed milk.
Since whole milk has a higher density than espresso, the latter will be placed above the milk.
Serve in a tumbler type glass.
To serve, you can fill the milk foam with chocolate flakes, liquid caramel, cocoa powder, cinnamon or other spices.

Nutrition

Calories: 80   Fat: 5 g
Carbohydrates: 5 g   Protein: 3 g

110. Latte Macchiato Caramel

Preparation Time: 15 minutes

Cooking Time: 0 minutes

Servings: 6

Ingredients

1 l of milk   20 cl of coffee
10 cl of caramel syrup

Directions

Make the recipe "Latte Macchiato Caramel" in the pan.
Heat the milk and prepare 20 cl of hot black coffee. Divide the milk into 4 large glasses and froth the milk with an emulsifier, electric whisk, or steam nozzle on your coffee maker until you have 2 to 3 cm of milk foam.
Pour about 2cl of caramel syrup into each glass and slowly pour 5cl of coffee.
The coffee will come just below the foam of milk, to form 3 layers: the milk at the bottom, the coffee, and the milk froth above.
Serve in a cup-type glass.
Pour a little caramel syrup over the milk foam.

Nutrition

Calories: 140   Fat: 5 g
Carbohydrates: 22 g   Protein: 2 g

111. Coffee Cream with Caramel Milk Foam

Preparation Time: 15 minutes

Cooking Time: 0 minutes

Servings: 4

Ingredients

Grand Cru Volluto capsule (to prepare 40 ml of Espresso coffee)
100 ml of milk to prepare milk foam
Teaspoon caramel syrup
25 ml / 5 teaspoons of cream (already prepared or homemade according to the method indicated below)

Ingredients for the preparation of 250 ml of homemade cream:
250 ml semi-skimmed milk   2 egg yolks
50 g of white sugar   Half vanilla pod cut lengthwise

Materials
Espresso Cup (80 Ml)   Recipe Spoon Ritual

Directions

Bring the milk to a boiling point along with half a vanilla pod in a casserole dish
Beat the egg yolks inside a bowl with the sugar
Continue beating the yolks and sugar while adding the milk with the half vanilla pod
Then, put the mixture back in the pan and let it thicken over low heat (do not let the mixture boil to prevent it from cutting)
Check the consistency of the cream with a spoon and, as soon as the cream begins to adhere to the spoon, remove the pan from the heat

Keep stirring the mixture to keep it soft and creamy
Take out the vanilla bean, scrape it with a knife to remove the seeds and put it back in the cream
Prepare a Volluto (25 ml) in an Espresso cup or a small Nespresso recipe glass and add 25 ml / five teaspoons of the homemade cream or ready-made cream
Prepare milk foam with the steam nozzle of your Nespresso machine or the Aeroccino milk frother and add the caramel syrup as soon as the foam begins to form
Cover the coffee cream with the caramel-flavored milk foam and serve immediately.

Nutrition

Calories: 26

Fat: 1.47 g

Carbohydrates: 2.91 g

Protein: 0.39 g

112. Hot and Cold Vanilla Espresso with Caramel Foam and Cookies

Preparation Time: 15 minutes

Cooking Time: 15 minutes

Servings: 4

Ingredients

For hot and cold vanilla coffee:
Two capsules of Grand Cru Volluto
A scoop of vanilla ice cream
Three tablespoons of milk foam
Two teaspoons of caramel liquid

For the cookies:

70 g softened butter	70 g of sugar
Teaspoon honey	Egg
100 g flour	A pinch of salt
50 g grated chocolate	

For hazelnut caramel:

50 g whole hazelnuts	40 g of sugar
Two tablespoons of water	

Directions

For hot and cold vanilla coffee:
Prepare the milk foam, add the liquid caramel, and reserve it.
Prepare two coffees in a large cup and pour them into a cold glass.
Add the vanilla ice cream ball immediately and cover it with the milk foam.

For cookies:
Preheat oven to 150 ° C
Heat sugar and water until caramelized, remove from heat and add crushed hazelnuts
Place the hazelnuts on a sheet of vegetable paper and roast them in the oven for 10 min, moving them occasionally
Put the butter, sugar, salt, honey and egg in a large bowl
Beat it all for a few seconds until you get a smooth mixture
Add caramelized hazelnuts and grated chocolate
Raise the oven temperature to 180 ° C
Put small balls of dough on the baking sheet lined with vegetable paper and bake for about 15 min
Let them cool on a rack

Nutrition . . . .

Calories: 190
Carbohydrates: 150 g

Fat: 11 g
Protein: .27 g

113. Espresso with Cottage Cheese, Lime and Brazil Nuts

Preparation Time: 5 minutes

Cooking Time: 20 minutes

Servings: 6

Ingredients

One capsule of Grand Cru Volluto or Volluto Decaffeinato

550 g cottage cheese   100 g of sugar

The juice of a lime   Two egg whites

Three jelly sheets   80 g of Brazil nuts

Directions

Roast the Brazil nuts in a pan and mash them finely. Book them. Dip the jelly leaves in cold water to soften them. Grate and squeeze the file.

Boil 100 ml of water with sugar and lime juice for 5 minutes. Remove from heat and add the drained gelatin and lime zest. Beat the egg whites and mount them until stiff.

Pour three-quarters of the lime syrup over the egg whites without stopping to beat and then add the cottage cheese to the mixture. Divide the crushed nuts into the six molds and cover them using a cottage cheese mousse.

Pour the remaining lime syrup over and put the molds in the refrigerator for 4 hours. Serve it with a Grand Cru Volluto.

Nutrition

Calories: 183   Fat: 5.31 g

Carbohydrates: 5.5 g   Protein: 27 g

114. Coffee with Malice

Preparation Time: 5 minutes

Cooking Time: 5 minutes

Servings: 4

Ingredients

One intense espresso coffee sachet   1 splash whiskey
1 splash whole milk or cream

Directions

You can use the dolce gusto machine, but if you don't have one, you can do it with a good quality soluble coffee loaded. All right; Put the coffee sachet in the coffee maker and select the amount of water to pour.
Activate the hot water until it stops. Have whiskey on hand. Pour a little squirt of whiskey, heat a little cream or milk, and add it to coffee.
Ready, you can add sugar or sweetener if it's your taste. I prefer it as it is. With its bitter touch.

Nutrition

Calories: 394   Fat: 9 g
Carbohydrates: 67 g   Protein: 10 g

115. Viennese coffee

Preparation Time: 5 minutes

Cooking Time: 0 minutes

Servings: 1

Ingredients

Espresso coffee to your liking
White sugar
Shavings chocolate

Whole milk
Whipped cream

Directions

Take the coffee capsule. You put it in the machine and let it do its job.

You fill the glass of milk, add your healthy dose of sugar, and stir.

Decorate with a good tuft of cream and chocolate chips.

As you can see, very, very difficult to do. Having just spent the day.

Nutrition

Calories: 251
Carbohydrates: 0.63 g

Fat: 27 g
Protein: 0.62 g

116. Coffee mousse

Preparation Time: 5 minutes

Cooking Time: 0 minutes

Servings: 6

Ingredients

4 sheets jelly
2 tablespoons. Baileys
Two egg whites

125 ml of espresso coffee
100 gr. sugar
200 ml 35% mg whipping cream

Directions

Put into hydrating the gelatin.
Prepare a coffee.
Ride the egg whites with the sugar about to snow.
Semi-cream.
Melt the jello in the hot coffee and add the Baileys.
Add the coffee to tablespoons to the whites mounted.
Add the whipped cream.
Pour the mixture into 6 glasses that you can decorate with sprinkled cocoa powder. In my case, I prepared a coffee jelly.
Let cool inside the fridge for a few hours and go!

Nutrition

Calories: 2
Carbohydrates: 4 g

Fat: 0.5 g
Protein: 0.28 g

Conclusion

Congratulations! You have made it to the end of this book! Are you convinced yet? We have gone over dozens of healthy, delicious recipes that look like they would be enjoyable for just about anyone, and even better, they are packed with sirtuins! Remember, there is no commitment—you do not have to commit to the calorie restrictions if you do not want to, but the recipes in this book are healthy and delicious for anyone.

Always remember that the sirtuins that you will be consuming will help you to keep your muscle mass up, and that is highly beneficial. Most diets will see you losing muscle mass, but when you make use of these Sirtfoods, you will find that there is surprising staying power for your muscles. Not only will it help you to hold on to the muscle that you already have, but you will also be seeing an increase of muscle as well.

Studies have shown that sirtuins can help boost muscle mass, especially in elderly individuals. A study done on aging mice showed that the sirtuin rich diet helped allow for the development and growth of blood vessels and muscle. This would then boost the energy that the elderly mice had by upwards of 80%. That is massive. If you want to make sure that your metabolism stays regulated, you must make sure that your muscles are there to help you, and if they are not, you can run into all sorts of problems. This means that if you really want to find a diet that will help you gain muscle and burn fat, the sirtuin-rich Sirtfood Diet may be one of the best for you.

If you are ready to tackle the Sirtfood Diet and are preparing to move on to phase one, congratulations! You can do it! Remember that all diets are a bit difficult at first. It takes weeks to form a new habit, and while you may miss the old foods, you will learn to love and crave the new ones just as quickly. If you want to be able to enjoy your diet and really thrive, losing any weight that you have to kick off and learning to create the healthy lifestyle that you need, this is the book for you.

Stick to it! You can do it! You've already taken a monumental step just in picking up this book to read in the first place. Now, if you are ready, go look up a juicer. Start putting together your meal plans and shopping lists. Get ready to go on the journey of a lifetime, losing weight and feeling better than ever before!

Thank you so much for choosing this book to guide you through your journey to healthiness and wellness— hopefully, you feel like you have made the right one! If you have enjoyed this book, please consider heading over to Amazon to leave a review with your experience. It would be greatly appreciated! Good luck on your journey, and know that you have the power to make these great changes if you want it!

CPSIA information can be obtained
at www.ICGtesting.com
Printed in the USA
BVHW041500180121
598054BV00006B/157